The UK Cardiology Curriculum: Joint Royal Colleges of Physicians Training Board (JRCPTB)

Azhar ul Haque Sario

Copyright

Azhar.sario@hotmail.co.uk

ORCID: https://orcid.org/0009-0004-8629-830X

LinkedIn: https://www.linkedin.com/in/azharulhaquesario/

Publisher Details Azhar Sario Hungary Author Website: www.linkedin.com/in/azharulhaquesario

Cataloging Data ISBN:

Google Version
978-3-384-80875-2

eBook Version
978-3-384-80876-9

Paperback Version
978-3-384-80877-6

First Edition: 2026 Printed & Distributed by PublishDrive

Contents

The Pedagogical Architecture of Modern Cardiology Training

2.0 The Strategic Shift: Shape of Training (SoT) and the Dual Mandate

2.1 The "Why" Behind the Change

To understand what you are learning, you must understand why the goalposts moved. The Shape of Training review was not an administrative shuffle; it was a survival strategy for the NHS.

The average patient admitted to a coronary care unit in 2026 is not a 50-year-old male with a single blocked artery. They are an 82-year-old female with non-ST elevation myocardial infarction (NSTEMI), Stage 3 chronic kidney disease, frailty, and mild cognitive impairment. The previous training model, which allowed cardiologists to shed their general medical skills early, created a workforce ill-equipped for this multi-morbid reality.

2.2 The Dual-Specialty Mandate

In the 2026 cycle, there is no "opt-out." Every cardiology trainee (Group 1 Specialty) is dual-accredited. You are training to be two consultants simultaneously:

A Consultant Cardiologist: Capable of high-level cardiac diagnostics and intervention.

A Consultant Physician in General Internal Medicine (GIM): Capable of running the acute unselected medical take.

The Functional Reality: This is not just about having two certificates. It means your rota will be a hybrid. You might spend Tuesday morning in the Cath Lab opening a blocked LAD artery, and Tuesday night on the medical registrar rota managing a patient with diabetic ketoacidosis or a GI bleed.

Course Note: This "dual mandate" significantly compresses the time available for pure cardiology. You have five years (ST4 to ST8) to master both. This requires a ruthless efficiency in your learning style, which we will discuss in the "Spiral Curriculum" section.

3.0 The Spiral Curriculum & Capability-Based Progression

The educational philosophy of the 2026 curriculum is the Spiral Model.

In linear learning, you learn a topic (e.g., "Pacing"), pass a test, and move on. In a spiral curriculum, you revisit the same themes repeatedly, but the complexity and your level of autonomy increase with each "turn" of the spiral.

3.1 The Trajectory of Entrustment

We no longer tick boxes to say you have "done" a procedure 50 times. instead, we ask: "Can you be trusted?"

Progress is measured by Capabilities in Practice (CiPs). These are high-level outcomes assessed by your supervisors. You will be rated on a 4-level scale of entrustment for each specific activity:

Level 1: You can observe (Entrusted to observe only).

Level 2: You can act with Direct Supervision (The consultant is scrubbed in next to you).

Level 3: You can act with Indirect Supervision (The consultant is in the coffee room or at home, but available by phone).

Level 4: You can act Unsupervised (You are the boss).

3.2 Case Study: Temporary Pacing

ST4 (Novice): You insert a temporary wire. Your registrar is holding your hand. (Level 2).

ST5 (Core): You insert the wire. The consultant is watching from the control room. (Level 2/3).

ST7 (Advanced): It is 3:00 AM. A patient has complete heart block. You insert the wire alone, check the threshold, and go back to bed. (Level 4).

The skill didn't change; the entrustment did.

4.0 The "Themes": Modular Specialization

Because the curriculum is compressed into five years, you cannot be an expert in everything. The "Jack of all trades" model is unsustainable for high-level intervention.

The 2026 curriculum forces a choice. You will maintain Core Cardiology skills throughout all five years, but from ST6 onwards, you will specialize in one of five Advanced Themes.

Theme A: Core Cardiology (The Foundation)

Status: Mandatory for everyone (ST4-ST8).

Scope: Heart failure management, basic arrhythmia handling, coronary care unit (CCU) leadership, and—crucially—Echocardiography.

The Echo Mandate: Every trainee must be competent in Transthoracic Echo (TTE). You cannot hide from this. By ST6, you should be able to scan a patient in shock and diagnose a tamponade or severe LV dysfunction immediately.

Theme B-F: The Advanced Modules

You will select one of the following to take to a "Level 4" (Consultant) standard:

Advanced Rhythm Management (EP & Devices): Complex ablation and implanting CRT/ICD devices.

Advanced Coronary Intervention (PCI): Stenting, angioplasty, and managing STEMIs.

Heart Failure: Advanced therapies, transplant assessment, and cardiomyopathy management.

Imaging: High-level Cardiac MRI (CMR), CT Coronary Angiography, and transoesophageal echo (TOE).

Adult Congenital Heart Disease (ACHD): Managing the growing population of adults surviving with congenital defects.

Strategic Advice: In 2026, "Imaging" is the fastest-growing module due to the explosion of CT coronary angiography in chest pain pathways. If you prefer non-invasive diagnostic puzzles over scrubbing in, this is your growth sector.

5.0 Assessment: How You Are Judged

The days of a single "exit exam" being the only hurdle are gone. You are under constant low-level surveillance through Workplace Based Assessments (WPBAs).

5.1 The Critical Tools

ACAT (Acute Care Assessment Tool): Used for GIM. A consultant reviews your decision-making on an acute take of 5+ patients. Did you prioritize correctly? Did you discharge safely?

DOPS (Direct Observation of Procedural Skills): Vital for the Cath Lab. You need these to move from Level 2 to Level 3 supervision in angiography or pacing.

MCR (Multiple Consultant Review): This is the most dangerous assessment if you are failing. It is not just one supervisor's opinion; it is the consensus of the entire department. "Is this trainee safe?"

5.2 The EECC (European Exam)

Yes, you still have to pass a big exam. The European Exam in Core Cardiology (EECC) is usually taken in ST5 or ST6. It is a knowledge-based hurdle. You cannot progress to your final years without it.

6.0 The Human Reality: "The Crisis of Time"

We must speak authentically about the friction in this system. The 2026 curriculum is ambitious. It asks you to be a General Medical Consultant and a Specialist Cardiologist in just five years.

The Tension: Many trainees find that 5 years is simply not enough time to gain the "muscle memory" required for complex procedures like PCI (stenting) while also doing General Medicine rotas.

The Result: Many trainees in the 2026 cohort are opting for "Post-CCT Fellowships." This means that after you finish your training and technically become a consultant, you might take an extra year (often abroad in Canada, Australia, or a high-volume UK center) to refine your hands-on skills before taking a permanent job.

This is not a failure of the trainee; it is a structural reality of the dual-training pathway.

1.3 The 2026 Recruitment Landscape and Entry Criteria

The ST4 Bottleneck: A Shift in Focus

In 2026, the transition from Internal Medicine Training (IMT) to Higher Specialty Training (ST4) remains the most competitive bottleneck in the UK medical career structure. However, the nature of the competition has shifted. It is no longer just about having the MRCP(UK) diploma—that is merely the ticket to the game. The real differentiator now is the granular evidence of clinical competence, specifically aligned with Internal Medicine Stage 1 (IMS1) outcomes.

The recruitment panels are looking for a specific type of doctor: one who can lead a cardiac arrest team at 3 AM, manage a septic patient with multi-organ failure, and safely run a busy medical take, all before they even touch a catheter or an echo probe.

The "Alternative Certificate": The Gateway for Non-Standard Applicants

For applicants who have not completed the standard UK Internal Medicine Training program (e.g., international graduates or those who took time out for research), the "Alternative Certificate to Enter Group 1 Higher Physician Specialty Training" is your lifeline. However, the 2026 iteration of this document is far more demanding than previous versions.

Key Change: Entrustment Levels In previous years, a supervisor could simply tick a box stating a trainee was "competent." The 2026 certificate requires specific evidence of entrustment levels for all Clinical Capabilities in Practice (CiPs).

Scenario Example: Imagine Dr. A, an applicant from overseas. Under the old system, her supervisor might have signed off that she is "competent in managing acute heart failure."

In the 2026 Certificate, the supervisor must explicitly rate her entrustment level. They must certify: "Dr. A is capable of managing acute heart failure unsupervised (Level 4)."

If the supervisor indicates she still requires "direct supervision" (Level 2) for managing acute kidney injury or sepsis, Dr. A would likely be ineligible for ST4 Cardiology, because the entry criteria demand Level 4 competence in all IMS1 Clinical CiPs. This ensures that a new ST4 registrar does not need "hand-holding" for general medical problems.

The "GIM-Ready" Standard: Unselected Medical Take

The most significant hurdle in the 2026 specifications is the requirement for experience in managing an "unselected medical take."

What does "unselected" mean? It means the patients you see are not filtered. You aren't just seeing chest pain patients in a coronary care unit. You are seeing the 90-year-old with a urinary tract infection, the diabetic with ketoacidosis, and the overdose patient.

The 2026 guidance emphasizes this because Cardiology is a dual-accreditation specialty. You will graduate as a Cardiologist and a General Physician. Therefore, recruitment panels screen for applicants who have already cut their teeth on the general medical frontline.

Clinical Example: Consider an applicant, Dr. B, who has spent the last two years working solely in a high-tech Tertiary Cardiac Centre. He is an expert at managing post-PCI complications but has not managed a simple pneumonia or a GI bleed in 24 months.

Under the 2026 criteria, Dr. B might struggle. The recruitment panel will scrutinize his application for evidence of maintaining general medical skills. If he cannot prove recent experience in managing the "unselected take"—perhaps by doing locum shifts in a

District General Hospital's Acute Medical Unit—he may be deemed unappointable, despite his cardiology knowledge.

The Merger of Evidence: Geriatrics and Critical Care

A subtle but vital change in the 2026 paperwork is the merging of the "Clinical Experience" and "Portfolio Evidence" sections. The recruiters now demand a "forensic" accounting of your time in two specific areas:

Geriatric Medicine: You must detail exactly where and when you gained experience managing frailty and multi-morbidity.

Critical Care: You need explicit evidence of managing Level 2/3 patients (e.g., those on inotropes or non-invasive ventilation).

Why this matters: The average cardiology patient in the UK is elderly with multiple comorbidities. A cardiologist who cannot manage a patient's co-existing delirium or renal failure is functionally incomplete.

1.4 The Structure of Specialization: Core vs. Advanced Themes

Once you successfully navigate the entry criteria, the training program itself is structured to prevent "premature specialization." The 2026 curriculum is strictly bifurcated into two phases.

Phase 1: Core Cardiology (ST4 – ST6)

The first two to three years are the "building block" years. The goal here is not to make you a world-class electrophysiologist, but to make you a safe, competent General Cardiologist.

During this phase, you are acquiring the Five Core Cardiology CiPs alongside the Eight Internal Medicine CiPs.

The Core Cardiology CiPs include:

Managing cardiac emergencies (e.g., STEMI, VT storm).

Managing stable cardiac conditions (e.g., chronic heart failure, stable angina).

Preventative cardiology and risk factor management.

Multi-disciplinary team working.

Basic procedural competence (e.g., angiography, pacing, echo).

Workforce Example: Dr. C is an ST5 trainee. Even though she eventually wants to be an interventionist, her rota involves covering the general cardiology ward, running rapid access chest pain clinics, and holding the "crash bleep" for the hospital. She is learning to manage the whole patient, not just the coronary artery. This breadth ensures that if she is the Consultant on-call in 10 years, she can handle anything that comes through the door.

Phase 2: Advanced Themes (ST6 – ST8)

The final phase involves high-intensity training in one of five specific modules. This is where you hone your sub-specialty craft.

The Five Advanced Themes:

Coronary Intervention: Complex PCI, rotablation, CTOs.

Cardiac Imaging: Advanced Echo, CMR, CT, Nuclear.

Arrhythmia Management: Electrophysiology studies and complex device implantation (ICDs/CRTs).

Adult Congenital Heart Disease (ACHD): Managing patients born with structural defects who are now surviving into adulthood.

Heart Failure: Advanced therapies, transplant assessment, mechanical support.

The "Critical Progression Point"

You cannot simply "drift" into an advanced theme. The transition, typically at ST6, is a hard gate known as a Critical Progression Point. To pass this gate, two things must happen:

EECC Exam: You must have passed the European Examination in Core Cardiology.

Level 3/4 Competence: You must be signed off as independent in all Core Cardiology CiPs.

Throttling and Workforce Planning: A unique feature of this modular system is the ability to "throttle" the number of trainees entering each theme based on NHS service needs.

Planning Example: In 2026, the NHS data shows a massive spike in heart failure admissions due to an aging population, but a saturation of interventional cardiologists.

The Deanery can decide to open 10 spots for the Heart Failure advanced theme but only 2 spots for Intervention. This prevents the system from training doctors for jobs that don't exist and ensures the workforce matches the actual patient demand. Trainees might have to compete for their preferred theme or adapt to the market needs.

Generic Professional Capabilities and Ethical Practice

1. Introduction: The Holistic Cardiologist in 2026

In the modern landscape of British medicine, the definition of a competent cardiologist has shifted. By 2026, technical dexterity in the catheter lab or precision in echocardiography is no longer enough. The Joint Royal Colleges of Physicians Training Board (JRCPTB) curriculum has evolved. It now places a massive, undeniable weight on the "soft" skills that actually make the "hard" science work.

We are looking at the Generic Capabilities in Practice (GPC). Specifically, we are examining Domain 1 and Domain 2. These cover professional behaviour and legal frameworks.

Why does this matter? Because a heart doesn't beat in a vacuum. It beats inside a person who has rights, fears, and legal protections. This coursework explores how a trainee must navigate the complex intersection of trust, law, and clinical excellence.

2. Professional Behaviour and Values (GPC Domain 1)

2.1 The Architecture of Trust

The curriculum identifies "Professional Behaviour and Trust" as the foundation of practice. This is not just about being polite to nurses or patients. It is a rigorous, assessable metric. In 2026, trust is a clinical tool. If a patient does not trust you, they will not take their medication. They will not agree to the angiogram.

The General Medical Council (GMC) establishes the baseline in Good Medical Practice. However, for a cardiology trainee, this goes deeper. It requires "functioning effectively within NHS systems."

What does this mean in reality? It means understanding that the NHS is a finite resource. A trainee cannot just order every test available. They must understand the cost, the waiting lists, and the management structures. They must be stewards of the system.

Example: Consider a trainee who wants to order a cardiac MRI for a patient with ambiguous symptoms. Professional behaviour involves checking the local guidelines. It involves speaking to the imaging team to prioritize urgency. It is not just demanding the scan; it is navigating the system to get the right test for the right patient without breaking the department's workflow.

2.2 The Duty of Candour: When Things Go Wrong

One of the most critical descriptors in this domain is the promotion of an "open and transparent culture." This is legally codified as the Statutory Duty of Candour.

In the high-pressure environment of cardiology, mistakes happen. A prescription might be delayed. A complication might occur during a PCI (Percutaneous Coronary Intervention). The "old school" approach might have been to hide these minor errors. The 2026 approach is radical transparency.

The curriculum demands that trainees possess the emotional intelligence to offer apologies. This is difficult. Doctors are trained to be right. Admitting you were wrong feels unnatural. But an apology is not an admission of legal liability in the way we often fear; it is a validation of the patient's experience.

Example: Imagine a patient's discharge summary was delayed, causing them to miss a dose of antiplatelets. A professional trainee does not blame the ward clerk. They go to the patient. They say, "I am sorry this happened. Here is exactly why it happened, and here is what I have done to ensure it doesn't happen to the next person." This rebuilds the trust that the error broke.

2.3 Social Determinants: Treating the Postcode, Not Just the Artery

Cardiovascular health is perhaps the medical field most heavily influenced by where and how a person lives. This is the "Social Determinants of Health."

The curriculum requires trainees to look beyond the biological. They must understand public health issues. In 2026, with the widening gap in health inequalities, this is vital. A patient from a deprived area is statistically more likely to smoke, have a poor diet, and suffer from hypertension.

If a cardiologist treats the myocardial infarction but ignores the fact that the patient cannot afford healthy food, the treatment has failed. The patient will return.

Example: A trainee treats a 50-year-old man for heart failure. The medical management is perfect. But the man lives in a damp, third-floor flat with no elevator. He cannot physically leave his home. His mental health deteriorates, and he stops taking his diuretics. A culturally competent trainee identifies this social barrier. They engage social services or occupational therapy before discharge. They treat the environment, not just the heart.

2.4 Measuring the Intangible: The MCR and MSF

How do we prove a trainee is "professional"? We cannot use a blood test.

We use the Multiple Consultant Report (MCR) and Multi-Source Feedback (MSF). These are the mirrors held up to the trainee.

MCR: Consultants discuss the trainee's integrity. Is she reliable? Does he call for help when drowning?

MSF: This is 360-degree feedback. Nurses, porters, and secretaries rate the trainee.

In 2026, the MSF is powerful. You can be the smartest doctor in the room, but if you are rude to the scheduling coordinator, you fail this domain. It ensures that "professionalism" is a consistent behaviour, not a mask worn only for the boss.

3. Legal Frameworks and Ethical Complexity (GPC Domain 2)

3.1 The Nuance of Capacity and Consent

The second Generic Capability in Practice (CiP) moves us into the courtroom of the mind. It deals with national legislation, specifically the Mental Capacity Act.

Cardiology is unique here. We often deal with patients who have lost capacity suddenly.

Cardiogenic Shock: The brain isn't getting enough oxygen. The patient is confused.

Cardiac Arrest: The patient is unconscious.

The trainee must be a master of the legal framework. They must understand the difference between a patient who makes a "bad" decision (which is their right) and a patient who cannot make a decision.

Example: A 75-year-old woman needs a TAVI (Transcatheter Aortic Valve Implantation). She refuses. The trainee must assess: Does she understand the risks? Can she retain the information? If she has early dementia, does she lack capacity? If she has capacity, the trainee must respect her refusal, even if it leads to death. Leading the team through this ethical minefield is a core skill.

3.2 End-of-Life Care and Device Deactivation

Technological advances have created new ethical dilemmas. We have devices that can keep a heart beating indefinitely. Implantable Cardioverter Defibrillators (ICDs) save lives. But at the end of life, they can cause unnecessary suffering.

Shocking a dying heart is cruel. The curriculum mandates that trainees can navigate the withdrawal of treatment. This includes the deactivation of ICDs.

This is an emotional discussion. The family often sees the device as a "life insurance" policy. Turning it off feels like "killing" the patient. The trainee must explain the legal and ethical shift from "preserving life" to "ensuring a dignified death."

Example: A patient with end-stage heart failure is moving to palliative care. He has an ICD. The trainee initiates the conversation early, perhaps weeks before the final days. They explain that the device will treat a fast rhythm but won't stop the heart from eventually stopping naturally. They arrange for the physiologists to deactivate the shock function while keeping the pacing function. This is a complex clinical, technical, and legal procedure managed entirely by the cardiologist.

3.3 Safeguarding: The Vulnerable Heart

Finally, the 2026 specifications highlight Safeguarding. This was once seen as the domain of paediatricians or GPs. No longer. Cardiologists treat the elderly, the frail, and those dependent on care.

We see patients when they are undressed. We see their bruising. We see who brings them to appointments—and who doesn't.

The curriculum requires trainees to identify signs of abuse or neglect. This could be physical abuse, or it could be financial abuse of a vulnerable adult.

Example: An elderly lady is admitted with heart failure decompensation. She appears malnourished. Her son, who is her carer, seems aggressive and insists she doesn't need her medication because "it's too expensive." A trainee trained in GPC Domain 2 recognizes this red flag. They do not ignore it. They document it. They contact the hospital safeguarding lead. They realize that her heart failure is a symptom of neglect.

4. Deep Dive Analysis: The 2026 Context

4.1 The Evolution of "Professional Integrity"

In the 2026 recruitment person specification, "Professional Integrity" is an essential selection criterion. Why is this emphasized so heavily now?

It is because the medical landscape has become transparent. Patients have access to their own records via apps. They can Google their symptoms. They can record consultations on their phones.

In this era, integrity is the only currency that matters. If a trainee tries to bluff their way through an explanation, they will be caught. If they try to hide a risk, it will be discovered.

The 2026 curriculum recognizes that a cardiologist acts as a team leader. If the leader lacks integrity, the team fractures. If the leader is defensive, the team hides errors.
4.2 Risk Minimization as a Competency

The specification also lists the "ability to minimize risk." This connects Domain 1 and Domain 2.

Risk minimization is not just about steady hands during surgery. It is about systems thinking.

It is the ethical choice to speak up if you are too tired to operate safely (Domain 1).

It is the legal requirement to ensure consent is valid so you don't perform the wrong procedure (Domain 2).

The modern trainee is a risk manager. They constantly scan the horizon for threats—clinical, legal, and social—and mitigate them before they become disasters.

Part 1: Communication and Shared Decision Making (Generic CiP 3)

Beyond "Soft Skills"

For decades, communication was viewed as a "soft skill." It was secondary to the "hard skills" of interpreting echoes or navigating catheters. The current curriculum rejects this dichotomy.

Communication is now a high-level clinical competency. It is graded with the same rigour as procedural skills. In the Coronary Care Unit (CCU), clear communication saves lives. Ambiguity causes errors.

The 2026 standard requires a sophisticated approach. The trainee must adapt to the audience. This is not just about being polite. It is about the precise transfer of information in high-stakes environments.

Example: Consider a cardiac arrest team leader. They do not need "polite" conversation. They need "closed-loop" communication. The leader instructs, "Give 1mg Adrenaline." The nurse confirms, "1mg Adrenaline given." This is a technical skill. The curriculum demands evidence of this precision.

Barriers to Understanding

A core component of Generic CiP 3 is the management of barriers. Patients in cardiology often face significant challenges. They may be elderly. They may have cognitive impairment due to vascular disease. They may face language barriers.

The trainee must identify these hurdles immediately. Ignorance is not a defence. If a patient does not understand their medication due to a language deficit, and they are readmitted with heart failure, that is a failure of clinical care, not just communication.

Example: A patient with early dementia is prescribed Warfarin. The biological decision is correct. However, the communication barrier (memory loss) means the patient cannot manage the dosing monitoring. A "competent"

cardiologist identifies this barrier. They switch to a Direct Oral Anticoagulant (DOAC) or arrange blister packing. They prioritize adherence over pure pharmacology.
The Deep Dive: Shared Decision Making (SDM)

The most significant pedagogical shift is "Shared Decision Making." This moves medicine away from Paternalism.

Paternalism is the "Doctor knows best" model. In that model, the doctor chooses the treatment and tells the patient. SDM is different. It is a partnership. The doctor brings the expertise on treatment. The patient brings the expertise on their life.

The curriculum aligns this with the legal standard set by the Montgomery ruling. This legal precedent established that we must tell patients what they would find significant, not just what we think is significant.

The TAVI vs. SAVR Paradigm: The curriculum frequently cites the choice between Transcatheter Aortic Valve Implantation (TAVI) and Surgical Aortic Valve Replacement (SAVR). This is the ultimate SDM exam question.

The Science: SAVR might have better long-term durability data. TAVI is less invasive but has vascular access risks.

The Patient: An 80-year-old patient might value a quicker recovery time (TAVI) over 20-year durability. They want to attend a granddaughter's wedding in three months.

The Competency: The trainee must explain the "risk-benefit ratio." They must explain stroke risk versus recovery time. They must do this without using medical jargon. Then, they must bow to the patient's values. If the patient chooses the "medically inferior" option because it aligns with their life goals, the doctor supports that choice. That is Generic CiP 3 in action.

The Multidisciplinary Team (MDT)

Communication is not strictly doctor-patient. It is also doctor-doctor and doctor-nurse. The curriculum mandates effective interaction within the MDT.

Cardiology is team-based. Heart Teams decide on complex revascularization. Endocarditis Teams manage infection. The trainee must demonstrate "situational awareness."

They must know when to speak up and when to listen. They must be able to present a case concisely to a room of surgeons, geriatricians, and anaesthetists. They must defend their clinical reasoning without being aggressive.

Example: A Registrar presents a case at the Valve MDT. The surgeon wants to operate. The Registrar notes the patient has severe frailty, identified by the bedside nurses. The Registrar advocates for the patient's likely inability to survive rehabilitation. This requires professional courage. It demonstrates the synthesis of clinical data and communication to influence the team decision.

Part 2: Research, Scholarship, and Data Management (Generic CiP 5)

The Academic-Vocational Hybrid

The UK Cardiology Curriculum is unique. It is a vocational programme; it trains you to do a job. But it is also an academic programme; it trains you to think like a scientist.

Generic CiP 5 mandates that all cardiologists must be research-literate. This does not mean everyone must be a Professor. It means everyone must understand the language of evidence.

There is a distinction between "doing research" and "applying research." The curriculum demands the latter as a baseline and encourages the former as excellence.

Critical Appraisal and Methodologies

Trainees must understand the machinery of truth. They must know the difference between a Randomized Controlled Trial (RCT) and an Observational Registry.

They need to understand statistical power. They must spot bias. In 2026, the volume of medical literature is overwhelming. A cardiologist cannot read everything. They must filter.

Example: A new drug is released for Heart Failure. The pharmaceutical rep claims a "50% relative risk reduction." The competent trainee asks, "What was the absolute risk reduction?" If the absolute reduction is 0.1%, the drug may not be worth the cost or side effects. This ability to deconstruct marketing using statistical principles is a core requirement of CiP 5.

Translating Research into Practice

This is the "implementation gap." Research takes years to happen. It takes even longer to reach the bedside. The curriculum requires trainees to bridge this gap.

They must apply Evidence-Based Medicine (EBM) to individual scenarios. Guidelines give general rules. Patients are specific exceptions.

Example: Guidelines say "Give Dual Antiplatelet Therapy (DAPT) for 12 months after a heart attack." Your patient has a high bleeding risk and a history of gastric ulcers. The "Research Competent" trainee looks for evidence on "Shortened DAPT duration." They find recent trials suggesting 3 months of DAPT is safe for high-bleed risk patients. They apply this specific evidence to deviate from the general guideline safely. This is high-level scholarship.

Data Management and Ethics

In 2026, data is the new blood. We manage terabytes of imaging data and genetic sequencing. CiP 5 covers the ethical management of this data.

Trainees must understand GDPR and patient confidentiality in the digital age. They must understand the ethics of consent. If you are recruiting a patient for a trial during a heart attack (acute setting), how do you get valid consent?

The curriculum requires knowledge of "Good Clinical Practice" (GCP). This is the international ethical and scientific quality standard for designing and conducting trials.

The 2026 Recruitment Context

The prompt specifically references the 2026 recruitment cycle. This is a competitive arena. The curriculum sets the minimum standard. Recruitment looks for the maximum standard.

"Desirable Criteria" often become de facto "Essential Criteria" due to competition.

The Baseline: Understanding research (CiP 5).

The Differentiator: "Exceptional achievement." This means high-impact publications. It means presenting at the European Society of Cardiology (ESC) or the American Heart Association (AHA).

Quality Improvement (QI): It is not just about discovering new science. It is about improving current systems. Trainees must show they have led a project that improved patient care.

Example of Differentiation: Candidate A has read the guidelines on Heart Failure. (Meets Curriculum). Candidate B conducted an audit on Heart Failure discharge summaries, found a deficit in coding, implemented a new checklist, and re-audited to show a 20% improvement in follow-up rates. (Exceeds Curriculum - Highly Competitive).

The Internal Medicine Interface and Acute Care

3.1 Managing the Acute Unselected Take (IM CiP 1)

The Philosophy of the "Unselected" Patient

The defining feature of the Group 1 specialty curriculum—which places Cardiology alongside Acute Medicine, Respiratory, and Geriatrics—is the requirement to manage the acute unselected take. This is not merely a logistical duty; it is a fundamental clinical capability.

"Unselected" implies the highest level of diagnostic uncertainty. Unlike a patient referred to a cardiology clinic with "palpitations" (where the pre-test probability of cardiac disease is high), the unselected patient presents with undifferentiated symptoms: "collapse," "breathlessness," or "confusion."

IM Clinical CiP 1 mandates that trainees demonstrate professional behavior and robust clinical reasoning when managing these patients. The scope is comprehensive, covering the entire patient journey from the moment of admission to discharge or transfer.

Clinical Reasoning Beyond the Heart

To function effectively on the acute take, the cardiologist must step outside the catheter lab and the echo room. The curriculum requires competence in managing conditions that may mimic cardiac disease or coexist with it.

Clinical Insight: Consider a patient presenting with hypotension and tachycardia. The "Cardiology Brain" looks for cardiogenic shock or tamponade. The "IM CiP 1 Brain" must simultaneously evaluate for sepsis (distributive shock), gastrointestinal bleeding (hypovolemic shock), or adrenal crisis.

Trainees must exhibit the ability to formulate differential diagnoses and management plans that account for patient preferences and urgency. This includes high-stakes decision-making in:

Sepsis: Rapid identification of the septic six, differentiating septic cardiomyopathy from primary cardiac failure.

Acute Kidney Injury (AKI): Managing fluid balance where the treatment for the kidney (hydration) conflicts with the heart (diuresis).

Respiratory Failure: Differentiating COPD exacerbations from pulmonary oedema—a classic "unselected" dilemma.

Neurological Emergencies: Managing acute stroke thrombolysis or recognising seizures that present as syncope.

Operational Competence and Workforce Resilience

The 2026 curriculum emphasizes that clinical skills alone are insufficient; operational competence is vital. Managing the "take" involves leading a multidisciplinary team, triaging scarce resources (like High Dependency Unit beds), and making safe discharge decisions.

By the end of training (ST7/ST8), the trainee must be entrusted to manage the acute take unsupervised (Level 4 Entrustment). This means they can effectively function as a Consultant Physician, taking full responsibility for the "medical registrar" list and the safety of the hospital at night. This requirement ensures the resilience of the acute medical workforce across the NHS, guaranteeing that a Consultant Cardiologist is not just a heart specialist, but a safe pair of hands for any medical emergency.

3.2 Management of Multi-Morbidity and Frailty (IM CiP 3)

The End of "Pure" Cardiology

As the population ages, "pure" cardiology patients—those with a single cardiac pathology and no other medical history—are becoming exceptionally rare. IM Clinical CiP 3 addresses the continuity of care for medical inpatients, specifically focusing on the management of comorbidities and cognitive impairment.

This subtopic requires trainees to recognize the dangerous interaction between cardiovascular disease and other physical or mental health conditions. A stent may fix a coronary artery, but it does not treat the patient's concomitant diabetes, renal impairment, or vascular dementia.

The Frailty Paradigm

The curriculum mandates competence in managing the frail older patient. Frailty is not just "getting old"; it is a distinct physiological state of reduced reserve. The 2026 curriculum requires cardiologists to become adept at:

Frailty Scoring: Using tools like the Clinical Frailty Scale (CFS) to guide decision-making.

Deprescribing: Recognising when "Guidelines Directed Medical Therapy" (GDMT) becomes a burden rather than a benefit. Managing complex polypharmacy is a key skill.

The "Ceiling of Care": Recognizing that aggressive cardiac interventions (like TAVI or complex PCI) may need to be balanced against quality of life and functional status.

Scenario: An 88-year-old female with severe aortic stenosis, moderate dementia, and a CFS score of 7 (Severely Frail).

Standard Cardiology Approach: Aortic valve replacement is indicated for prognosis.

IM CiP 3 Approach: A nuanced discussion involving Geriatrics. Will the procedure improve her quality of life? Is she at risk of post-operative delirium? Is conservative management more aligned with her preferences?

Integration with Other Specialties

IM CiP 3 necessitates appropriate liaison with other specialties (e.g., renal, diabetes, geriatrics). The "Cardio-Geriatric" meeting is becoming as important as the Heart Team meeting.

The 2026 recruitment criteria specifically highlight the need for experience in geriatric medicine. Applicants for ST4 Cardiology posts are now required to detail the duration and supervision of their geriatric attachments. This reflects the reality that a significant proportion of the acute take involves patients over 75 with multiple comorbidities. Evidence of managing delirium, falls, and continence issues is no longer "optional"—it is a core recruitment metric.

Deep Dive Analysis: The "Generalist" Shift

Why this Matters in 2026

The shift towards Group 1 dual accreditation acknowledges a systemic reality in the NHS. The siloed model of medicine is failing the modern patient. A patient admitted with Heart Failure is likely to also have COPD and Chronic Kidney Disease (CKD). If a cardiologist treats only the heart failure and ignores the COPD, the patient will bounce back into the hospital.

IM CiP 1 and 3 are the antidotes to "siloed" medicine. They force the specialist to zoom out.

In IM CiP 1 (Acute Take), the skill is Diagnostic Width. You must cast a wide net to ensure you don't miss non-cardiac pathology.

In IM CiP 3 (Frailty), the skill is Therapeutic Depth. You must understand the patient deeply enough to know when not to treat, or when to modify standard treatment to fit a frail physiology.

The Trainee Journey: ST4 to ST8

ST4 (Early Stage): The trainee is expected to lead the cardiac arrest team but may need support with complex septic shock or status epilepticus on the medical take. They are learning to balance the "Specialty" view with the "Generalist" view.

ST6 (Mid Stage): The trainee begins to manage the "take" with distant supervision. They are comfortable managing a "medical outlier" on the cardiology ward who develops hospital-acquired pneumonia.

ST8 (Final Stage): The trainee achieves Level 4 Entrustment. They are rota-ed to lead the acute medical take independently. They can troubleshoot a busy AMU, support the IMT doctors, and make high-level decisions on escalation and palliation without needing to call the medical consultant on call.

3.3 Outpatient and Community Interfaces (IM CiP 4)

The Art of De-Escalation and Sustainability

The hospital is a high-intensity environment, but 99% of a patient's life is lived outside it. IM CiP 4 is about ensuring that the care we initiate in the hospital is sustainable when the patient returns home. It forces us to ask: "Is this plan realistic for a 75-year-old living alone?"

1. The Evolution of the Outpatient Clinic (2026 Perspective) By 2026, the outpatient clinic has transformed. It is no longer just a conveyor belt of face-to-face 15-minute slots. It is a hybrid ecosystem.

The Hybrid Model: Trainees must now demonstrate competence in triaging which patients need physical examination (e.g., a new murmur) versus those better served by high-definition video consultation (e.g., heart failure symptom review).

The "One-Stop" Philosophy: To respect the patient's time and reduce hospital footfall, we aim for the "one-stop" clinic. A patient with stable angina shouldn't come on Monday for an ECG, Tuesday for a blood test, and Thursday for a review. In 2026, we coordinate these into a single, high-value interaction.

2. The "Actionable" GP Letter The most critical skill in CiP 4 is communication with Primary Care. The General Practitioner (GP) is the conductor of the patient's orchestra; the cardiologist is merely a guest soloist.

The Failure of "Update Only": A letter that simply says "Patient seen, doing well, see you in 6 months" is a failure. It wastes the GP's reading time.

The Gold Standard (2026): Letters must be actionable. They must guide the GP on specific triggers.

Example: Instead of "Monitor BP," write: "Please titrate Ramipril to 10mg if systolic BP remains >130mmHg and renal function is stable. If creatinine rises >20%, please revert to 5mg."

This empowers the community team to act without sending the patient back to the Emergency Department.

3. Chronic Condition Management: The Big Three The curriculum highlights three pillars where community interface is vital:

Hypertension: This is the silent killer managed almost entirely in the community. The trainee's role is to investigate secondary causes (like Conn's syndrome) in resistant cases, but then hand back control to the GP with a clear roadmap. We don't hoard patients; we empower the community to manage them.

Heart Failure (HF): In 2026, "Hospital at Home" is standard. Patients with decompensated HF are increasingly treated in their living rooms with IV diuretics delivered by community heart failure nurses. The trainee must know how to govern this "virtual ward"—reviewing weight charts and renal function remotely and adjusting doses without a hospital bed.

Stable Angina: The focus has shifted from "plumbing" (stenting everything) to "prevention." The trainee must construct a lifestyle and pharmacological plan (statins, anti-anginals) that the patient can actually stick to. If a patient can't afford their prescription or doesn't understand why they are taking it, the plan has failed.

4. Preventing the Revolving Door The ultimate metric of success for CiP 4 is readmission prevention.

Scenario: Mr. Singh is discharged with Heart Failure.

Poor Practice: He is given a bag of pills and a follow-up in 3 months. He runs out of Furosemide in 3 weeks, retains fluid, and is readmitted.

CiP 4 Mastery: The trainee ensures Mr. Singh has a "sick day rule" card (e.g., "If weight goes up by 2kg, take an extra tablet"), a confirmed appointment with the community HF team within 48 hours, and a discharge summary sent to his GP immediately.

3.4 Resuscitation and End-of-Life Care (IM CiP 7 & 8)
The Spectrum of Intervention

This subtopic deals with the most profound decisions a doctor can make: when to fight for life with every technological tool available (CiP 7), and when to pivot to ensuring a peaceful, dignified death (CiP 8).
IM CiP 7: Resuscitation and the Acute Deterioration

"The Golden Hour"

Cardiology trainees are the natural leaders of the cardiac arrest team. However, CiP 7 goes beyond just knowing the algorithms of Advanced Life Support (ALS). It is about situational awareness.

1. The Deteriorating Patient Before the cardiac arrest, there is almost always a period of deterioration. The "crash" is rarely sudden; it is usually signaled by a drift in physiology.

Recognition: The trainee must spot the "pre-arrest" patient—the one with the rising lactate, the drifting respiratory rate, or the subtle confusion.

The "A to E" Reflex: In 2026, despite all our AI monitoring tools, the clinical assessment remains king. Airway, Breathing, Circulation. A trainee must be able to walk into a chaotic room, silence the noise, and methodically assess these three priorities.

2. Leadership in Chaos During a cardiac arrest, the trainee is the "Team Leader." This is a non-technical skill.

The Huddle: It's about assigning roles clearly. "You are on airway. You are on drugs. I am time-keeping."

Cognitive Offloading: A good leader doesn't touch the patient. They stand back, watch the monitor, watch the team, and think about the reversible causes (The 4 Hs and 4 Ts). If you are doing chest compressions, you cannot think about the diagnosis.

IM CiP 8: Managing End-of-Life

"The Shift to Palliative Care"

This is perhaps the most challenging aspect of modern cardiology. We have become so good at keeping people alive that we sometimes forget how to let them die. IM CiP 8 mandates that trainees recognize when the "battle" is changing.

1. The Prognostic Paralysis In cancer, the decline is often predictable. In Heart Failure, it is a roller-coaster—dips and recoveries, dips and recoveries—until one day, there is a dip from which there is no recovery.

The Skill: The trainee must identify "limited reversibility." When a patient is on their fourth admission for pulmonary oedema in three months, and their kidneys are failing, another round of IV diuretics might not be the answer.

The Conversation: This requires a high-level communication skill. It is not "giving up"; it is "reframing hope." We move from hoping for a cure to hoping for a comfortable, symptom-free conclusion.

2. The DNACPR Decision Discussion of "Do Not Attempt Cardiopulmonary Resuscitation" (DNACPR) is a core competency.

2026 Context: We have moved away from paternalism ("I am deciding this") to shared understanding ("Let's discuss what CPR actually involves").

Authentic Communication: Trainees must explain that CPR is a brutal, traumatic intervention designed for reversible events (like a VF arrest in a fit person), not a dying process for a frail heart.

Example phrasing: "I worry that if your heart were to stop, it would be because your body is too tired to go on. In that situation, CPR would not restart your heart, but it would deprive you of a peaceful ending with your family."

3. Symptom Control in Cardiac Death Palliative care in cardiology is different from oncology.

Breathlessness (Dyspnoea): This is the terrifying symptom of end-stage heart failure. The trainee must be confident in prescribing opioids (like morphine) not just for pain, but for air hunger.

Anxiety: The fear of drowning (pulmonary oedema) is real. The judicious use of benzodiazepines (like Lorazepam) is a compassionate act of medical care.

Deactivating Devices: By 2026, many patients have ICDs (defibrillators). A trainee must remember to deactivate the "shock" function of an ICD in a dying patient. There is nothing more tragic than a patient receiving a painful electric shock moments before death.

Core Theme: Coronary Artery Disease and Intervention

4.1 Acute Coronary Syndromes (ACS) Management

The Acute Presentation: Assessment and Instigation

The first hour of an ACS presentation is the "Golden Hour." Your ability to assess, investigate, and instigate management here defines patient survival. In 2026, the reliance on high-sensitivity troponins has been refined by rapid rule-in/rule-out algorithms (0/1-hour protocols) which are now standard across almost all NHS Trusts.

Assessment Protocols: You must be able to differentiate the chest pain that kills from the chest pain that annoys. This starts with the 12-lead ECG. But it goes beyond ST-elevation. You must recognize the subtle signs: the hyperacute T-waves, the De Winter T-waves, or the reciprocal changes in aVR that suggest left main stem disease.

Clinical Scenario: A 55-year-old diabetic male presents with "indigestion" and breathlessness. His ECG shows no ST elevation but widespread ST depression.

Action: You recognize this isn't just NSTEMI; it could be multi-vessel disease. You instigate dual antiplatelet therapy (DAPT) immediately but hold the P2Y12 inhibitor if you suspect urgent CABG might be needed. This is the level of nuance required.

Coordination of the PPCI Service

The Primary Percutaneous Coronary Intervention (PPCI) pathway is the jewel in the crown of UK cardiology. As a trainee, you are the conductor of this orchestra.

You might not be the one inflating the balloon (unless you are an intervention trainee), but you control the flow. You take the call from the paramedic. You decide if the patient bypasses A&E to go straight to the Cath Lab.

Logistical Mastery:

The Activation: You receive a pre-alert. You clear the lab. You brief the physiologist and nurses.

The "Door-to-Balloon" Time: You are responsible for minimizing delays. Every minute of delay is muscle lost.

Managing "False" Activations: Not every ST-elevation is an MI. You must be prepared to manage pericarditis, Takotsubo cardiomyopathy, or aortic dissection mimicking STEMI.

Pharmacotherapy: The 2026 Standard

The drug regimen for ACS has evolved. We have moved away from "one size fits all."

Anti-platelets: Aspirin remains the anchor. But the second agent is the variable.

Ticagrelor/Prasugrel: These are the standards for ACS.

De-escalation: By 2026, guided de-escalation (switching from potent agents like Prasugrel to Clopidogrel after the acute phase) is common, often guided by genotype testing or platelet function tests to reduce bleeding risk without losing ischaemic protection.

Anti-coagulants: In the cath lab, Unfractionated Heparin (UFH) or Bivalirudin are king. On the ward for NSTEMI, Fondaparinux is the standard due to its safety profile.

Example: A patient with high bleeding risk (e.g., previous ulcer, elderly) comes in with STEMI. The protocol suggests Prasugrel. You, using clinical judgment, might opt for Clopidogrel or a lower dose of Ticagrelor. This deviation from protocol, based on patient safety, marks the transition from novice to expert.

Managing Complications

ACS is not always smooth sailing. The myocardium can fail.

Cardiogenic Shock: This is the highest mortality state. It requires rapid decision-making regarding mechanical circulatory support (MCS).

Impella vs. IABP: While the Intra-Aortic Balloon Pump (IABP) has fallen out of favor for routine use, micro-axial flow pumps (like Impella) or ECMO (Extracorporeal Membrane Oxygenation) are utilized in specialist centers for profound shock.

The Trainee Role: You must stabilize the patient with inotropes (Noradrenaline/Dobutamine) and coordinate transfer to a shock center if your hospital lacks MCS capabilities.

Mechanical Complications: These are catastrophic.

Ventricular Septal Defect (VSD): A harsh new murmur post-MI.

Papillary Muscle Rupture: Sudden pulmonary oedema and a murmur.

Free Wall Rupture: Usually results in tamponade and PEA arrest.

Diagnosis: Urgent Echo is mandatory.

Management: These are surgical emergencies. Your role is to keep the patient alive (often requiring intubation and supports) while the surgeons prepare.

4.2 Stable Ischaemia and Risk Factor Modification

The Diagnostic Shift: CT First

The era of the diagnostic angiogram for everyone is over. The UK guidelines (NICE) and ESC guidelines have firmly placed CT Coronary Angiography (CTCA) as the first-line investigation for stable chest pain.

Why CT? It is non-invasive and has a high negative predictive value. If the CT is normal, you can discharge the patient with confidence.

Functional Testing: When the CT shows "moderate" disease, or calcium bloom makes it unreadable, we turn to functional testing.

Stress Echo: Great for assessing valve function alongside ischaemia.

Perfusion Scans (MPS/MRI): excellent for viability. If a patient has a chronic total occlusion (CTO), is the muscle alive? MRI answers this.

Example: A 60-year-old female with atypical pain has a CT showing a calcified LAD stenosis. You don't rush to angio. You order a Stress MRI. It shows no ischaemia. You treat medically. You have saved her an invasive procedure and a stent she didn't need.

INOCA: The Invisible Disease

For decades, if the angiogram was clear, patients were told "it's not your heart." We now know this was wrong. Ischaemia with Non-Obstructive Coronary Arteries (INOCA) is a major focus in 2026.

The Mechanism: It is often microvascular dysfunction (the tiny vessels don't dilate) or vasospastic angina (the vessels clamp shut).

Management:

Diagnosis: In the cath lab, we now use pressure wires not just for FFR (flow reserve) but to measure IMR (Index of Microcirculatory Resistance).

Treatment: Beta-blockers might worsen vasospasm. Calcium channel blockers and nicorandil become the heroes here. Recognizing INOCA validates the patient's symptoms and improves quality of life.

Refractory Angina

What do you do when the plumbing is fixed, or cannot be fixed, and the patient still has pain? This is refractory angina.

The Toolbox:

Optimized Medical Therapy: pushing anti-anginals to the max (Ranolazine, Ivabradine).

Enhanced External Counterpulsation (EECP): A non-invasive therapy growing in use.

Neuromodulation: Spinal cord stimulators for pain control (though rare).

Psychological Support: Chronic pain wears people down. Acknowledging the psychological burden is part of the treatment.

Preventative Cardiology: The Long Game

You cannot fix coronary disease; you can only manage it. The real battle is prevention.

Lipids: The "Lower is Better" Mantra: By 2026, the targets for LDL-cholesterol are aggressive. For secondary prevention (post-MI), we aim extremely low (<1.4 mmol/L or even lower).

Statins: High-intensity statins are just the start.

Ezetimibe: Added early.

PCSK9 Inhibitors/Inclisiran: These injectable agents are now introduced much earlier in the pathway for high-risk patients. Inclisiran, the "vaccine for cholesterol" (given every 6 months), has revolutionized adherence.

Hypertension: The silent killer. We now focus on ambulatory monitoring to catch "masked" hypertension. The target is strict control to prevent the shear stress that ruptures plaques.

Cardiac Rehabilitation: This is not an optional extra. It is a Class I indication. It reduces mortality. Your job is to "prescribe" rehab just as you prescribe aspirin. You must explain to the patient that exercise, diet, and smoking cessation are as powerful as the stent.

Deep Dive Analysis: The 2026 Perspective

As we look at the state of cardiology in the UK in 2026, several key themes emerge that differentiate current practice from a decade ago.

1. The Rise of Artificial Intelligence in Imaging AI is no longer sci-fi. It is in the scanner. When a patient has a CTCA, AI algorithms now auto-quantify plaque burden and even predict FFR (CT-FFR) without an invasive wire. This helps trainees make faster, more accurate decisions about who needs the cath lab.

2. Poly-pharmacy Management Patients are older and have more comorbidities. The skill of a cardiologist is now often deprescribing. Do they really need the proton pump inhibitor long-term? Can we stop the beta-blocker one year post-MI if LV function is normal? Rationalizing medication is a key safety skill.

3. The "Inflammatory" Hypothesis We are treating inflammation as a risk factor. High-sensitivity CRP is watched. Drugs like Colchicine (low dose) are increasingly used in chronic coronary syndromes to dampen the inflammatory fire that drives plaque instability.

4. Patient-Centric Decision Making The paternalistic "doctor knows best" is gone. We use Shared Decision Making aids. Does the 85-year-old with stable angina want

a stent, or does he just want to be able to walk to the shops without breathlessness? If pills achieve that, we skip the stent. The curriculum demands you document these discussions.

Section 1: 4.3 Invasive Angiography Skills

The Core Competency Requirement

Invasive coronary angiography remains the gold standard for defining coronary anatomy. Despite the rise of CT coronary angiography (CTCA), the ability to invasively interrogate the coronary tree is a non-negotiable skill for the core cardiology curriculum.

By the time you reach ST6, the expectation differs depending on your chosen sub-specialty stream. However, the foundational requirement is universal: safety, interpretation, and vascular competence.

For trainees pursuing the Intervention Stream, the target is clear. You must achieve Level 3 or Level 4 competence.

Level 3: You are able to perform the procedure independently but may need occasional advice from a supervisor who is available on-site.

Level 4: You are fully competent to perform the procedure independently without supervision.

For trainees in non-interventional streams (such as Imaging, Heart Failure, or Electrophysiology), the curriculum acknowledges that maintaining high-volume independent practice in diagnostic angiography may not be feasible or necessary for your consultant role.

The Derogation: Flexibility in Training

The 2022 curriculum (fully embedded by now in 2026) introduced a vital "derogation." This allows flexibility. If you are not an intervention trainee, you may exit training with Level 2 competence in invasive angiography.

Level 2: You can perform the procedure under limited supervision.

This derogation prevents the bottleneck of forcing heart failure specialists to compete for cath lab time just to tick a box. However, do not mistake this for an exemption. You must still understand the procedure intimately. You must be able to consent patients, recognize complications, and interpret the images for the European Examination in Core Cardiology (EECC).

Vascular Access: The 2026 Standard

The era of "femoral first" as a default is over. In 2026, radial access is the mandated standard of care for diagnostic angiography due to its superior safety profile regarding bleeding complications.

Competence in 4.3 requires you to master ultrasound-guided radial puncture. This is no longer an "optional extra"; it is a core safety skill. You must demonstrate the ability to visualize the radial artery, identify anatomical variants (like a high bifurcation), and cannulate successfully with a micropuncture kit.

Example Scenario: Consider an elderly patient with calcified radial arteries. A Level 3 trainee does not just "try and fail." They assess the arm with ultrasound first. If the radial is occluded or too small (less than 2mm), they immediately switch to the distal radial or ulnar approach, or safely transition to the femoral route using a micropuncture needle and fluoroscopic guidance to prevent high sticks.

Hemodynamics and Catheter Skills

It is not enough to just inject dye. You must be competent in the independent insertion of arterial lines and central venous cannulae (CVCs).

Why is this linked to angiography? Because the cath lab is often the venue for right heart catheterization (RHC) and hemodynamic instability management. You must be comfortable placing a 6F sheath in the internal jugular vein or femoral vein to measure filling pressures during a complex diagnostic case.

You must also master catheter manipulation. You need to know which shape—Judkins, Amplatz, or Multipurpose—to reach for when a coronary ostium is anomalous or the aorta is dilated.

Managing Risks and Complications

The curriculum places heavy emphasis on the "peri-procedural" cognitive skills. You must be the safety barrier for the patient.

Contrast-Associated Acute Kidney Injury (CA-AKI): Formerly known as contrast nephropathy. You must be able to calculate the safe contrast volume limit (e.g., using the formula 5×Body Weight/Creatinine). In 2026, we focus heavily on hydration status pre-procedure. You need to verify if the patient is on SGLT2 inhibitors (which should be paused) or nephrotoxic agents.

Vascular Complications: You must know how to manage a radial artery spasm (using verapamil/nitrates) and how to diagnose a retroperitoneal bleed if femoral access was used. If a patient becomes hypotensive post-procedure, your first instinct should not be "fluids" alone, but an urgent assessment of the access site.

Section 2: 4.4 Special Populations in Coronary Disease

This section moves beyond the standard "middle-aged male with angina" to complex, high-stakes patient groups. The curriculum demands that you act as a consultant-level resource for other specialties.

Coronary Disease in Pregnancy

Managing heart disease in pregnancy is one of the highest-pressure environments in cardiology. The 2025 ESC Guidelines on Cardiovascular Disease in Pregnancy have reshaped how we approach this.

Risk Stratification (mWHO 2.0): You must be fluent in the modified World Health Organization (mWHO) classification.

mWHO I: Low risk (small VSD, repaired PDA).

mWHO IV: Pregnancy contraindicated (e.g., Pulmonary Arterial Hypertension, severe reduced LV function <30%).

Spontaneous Coronary Artery Dissection (SCAD): In 2026, we recognize SCAD as the most common cause of pregnancy-associated myocardial infarction (PAMI). It often occurs in the immediate post-partum period.

The curriculum requires you to recognize the subtle signs: a healthy post-partum woman with "indigestion" or chest pain. You must know that invasive angiography carries a risk of propagating the dissection. Therefore, the decision to catheterize is weighty. If you do catheterize, you must be extremely gentle. Conservative management (beta-blockers, healing) is often preferred over stenting unless there is ongoing ischemia.

The Pregnancy Heart Team: You cannot work in a silo. The "Pregnancy Heart Team" concept is now standard. This team includes a cardiologist, an obstetrician, an anesthetist, and a neonatologist. Your role is to liaise effectively. You must draft a delivery plan by 32 weeks gestation that details:

Mode of delivery (Vaginal is usually preferred for cardiac patients to avoid surgical stress, unless there is severe aortic pathology).

Fluid management (avoiding auto-transfusion volume overload post-delivery).

Analgesia (early epidural to reduce cardiac stress).

Example Scenario: A 34-year-old woman at 28 weeks gestation presents with chest pain. Troponin is elevated. A standard trainee might rush to the cath lab. A competent ST6 trainee pauses. They perform a bedside echo first to look for wall motion abnormalities. They shield the abdomen. They discuss with the obstetric team about fetal monitoring during the angiogram. They use the radial approach to minimize radiation to the fetus.

Non-Cardiac Surgery and Peri-Operative Care

The cardiologist is frequently called to the pre-assessment clinic or the surgical ward. "Clearance for surgery" is an outdated term. We now provide Risk Assessment and Optimization.

Peri-operative Ischemia: The stress of surgery triggers a catecholamine surge, increasing myocardial oxygen demand. You must be able to assess this risk using tools like the RCRI (Revised Cardiac Risk Index) or newer biomarkers.

Biomarker Surveillance (MINS): We now actively look for "Myocardial Injury after Non-cardiac Surgery" (MINS). This involves checking Troponin levels 48-72 hours post-major surgery in high-risk patients. You must distinguish this from a Type 1 plaque rupture MI. MINS is often a supply/demand mismatch (Type 2 MI) and is treated with optimization of heart rate and blood pressure, rather than rushing to stents.

Antiplatelet Management: A core skill is managing the "Stent vs. Surgery" dilemma.

If a patient has a recent Drug-Eluting Stent (DES), elective surgery should ideally be delayed for 6 months.

If surgery is urgent (e.g., cancer resection), you may need to operate after 1-3 months with dual antiplatelet therapy (DAPT) maintained or bridged.

You must be the one to write the plan: "Continue Aspirin, stop Clopidogrel 5 days pre-op, restart 24 hours post-op if hemostasis is secure."

Liaison with Intensive Care: In the post-operative phase, patients may develop atrial fibrillation or heart failure. You are the resource for the ICU. You need to decide if the new hypotension is septic shock (low SVR) or cardiogenic (low output). A quick bedside echo or invasive line insertion (as detailed in section 4.3) might be the deciding factor.

Core Theme: Cardiac Imaging and Structural Disease

2.0 Assessment of Structural Heart Disease

Structural heart disease is the physical failure of the heart's architecture—the valves, the walls, and the great vessels. As a trainee, your primary role is detection, stabilisation, and pathway planning.

2.1 The "Front Door" Presentation: Murmurs, Syncope, and Emboli

You will often meet these patients on the acute medical take. They don't walk in with a diagnosis; they walk in with a story.

Syncope on Exertion: In 2026, this is a red flag that screams severe aortic stenosis (AS) until proven otherwise. With the release of the "Early TAVR" trial data in late 2024, our threshold for intervening has lowered. We no longer wait for severe heart failure. If they have syncope and severe AS, they are a structural emergency.

The "New" Murmur: You must differentiate the benign flow murmur from the sinister pathology. A harsh systolic murmur at the base? Think AS. A blowing diastolic murmur? Think Aortic Regurgitation (AR).

Real-world context: In the elderly, the murmur is often softer due to low flow states, even if the stenosis is critical. Do not trust your ears alone; trust the echo.

Embolic Phenomena: A young patient with a stroke and a fever is Infective Endocarditis (IE) until proven otherwise. You need to look for the classic signs—splinter haemorrhages, Janeway lesions—but these are rare. The real skill is knowing when to trigger the "IE Pathway."

2.2 The "Endocarditis Team" (MDT)

Managing Infective Endocarditis (IE) is no longer a solo sport. The 2023 and updated 2025 ESC guidelines solidified the mandate for an Endocarditis Team.

Who is on your team?

You (The Cardiologist): You own the echo and the haemodynamic assessment.

The Microbiologist: They are the guardians of the antibiotics. You will likely be prescribing high-dose regimens (e.g., flucloxacillin or vancomycin) that last 4-6 weeks.

The Cardiac Surgeon: They decide if and when to cut.

The ID Specialist: For complex multi-drug resistant organisms.

The "Timing" Dilemma: One of your hardest decisions in ST4/ST5 will be timing surgery in IE.

Too early? The tissues are friable and inflamed; the stitches might tear.

Too late? The patient might stroke out from a vegetation embolising to the brain.

The 2026 Standard: We now push for early surgery (within 48 hours) if there is heart failure, uncontrolled infection (persistent fever/positive cultures), or large vegetations (>10mm) with embolic events.

2.3 Anticoagulation and Valve Management

Valves are great, but they are thrombogenic. Managing the blood thinners is a core competency.

Mechanical Valves: Despite all our advances, Warfarin (Vitamin K Antagonist) remains the king here. DOACs (like Apixaban or Rivaroxaban) are still contraindicated for mechanical valves in 2026. You must manage the INR range strictness (usually 2.5–3.5 for mitral, 2.0–3.0 for aortic).

Bioprosthetic Valves & TAVI: Here, the landscape has changed. We often use a single antiplatelet (Aspirin) or a short course of anticoagulation depending on bleeding risk.

Pregnancy: This is a high-stakes exam topic and a real-life stress test. A pregnant woman with a mechanical valve needs a meticulous balance of LMWH (Low Molecular Weight Heparin) and Warfarin to protect the mother from thrombosis and the baby from teratogenicity.

3.0 Echocardiography Competence

If the stethoscope is the symbol of the past, the echo probe is the tool of the present. The curriculum is blunt: you cannot be a cardiologist if you cannot echo.

3.1 The "Workhorse" of Cardiology

Transthoracic Echocardiography (TTE) is the first-line test for almost everything. It is safe, portable, and gives instant haemodynamic data.

Physics in a nutshell: We use piezoelectric crystals to send ultrasound waves. They bounce off blood and tissue.

The time it takes to return tells us "depth," and the shift in frequency (Doppler) tells us "speed."

3.2 Level 1: Emergency Echo (The ST4 Requirement)

By the end of ST4, you must be competent in "Emergency Echo." This is a focused scan for the sickest patients. You are answering binary questions:

Is there a pericardial effusion? (Rule out Tamponade).

Is the LV working? (Rule out severe failure/shock).

Is the RV dilated? (Rule out massive Pulmonary Embolism).

Scenario: A patient arrives in resus with BP 70/40. You put the probe on. You see a swinging heart in a bag of black fluid (effusion) with a collapsed right atrium. Diagnosis: Tamponade. Action: Drain it. You saved a life before the bloods were even back.

3.3 Level 2: Full Competence (The BSE Standard)

By ST5, you need "Level 2" competence. This is usually evidenced by British Society of Echocardiography (BSE) accreditation. This is a massive undertaking involving:

Written Exam: Physics and pathology.

Logbook: 250 cases collected over 24 months.

Practical Exam: A grueling session where you scan a patient while an examiner watches your every hand movement.

What is the difference? Level 2 is quantitative. You aren't just saying "The leak is bad." You are measuring the PISA radius, the Vena Contracta, and the Pressure Half-Time. You are quantifying diastolic function to tell if the breathlessness is from the lungs or a stiff heart (HFpEF).

4.0 Deep Dive Analysis: The 2026 Landscape (New Information)

You asked for a deep dive into "new" information relevant to 2026. This is where the curriculum meets the cutting edge.

4.1 The Tricuspid Revolution

For decades, the tricuspid valve was the "forgotten valve." Surgeons hated touching it because patients did poorly.

The Change: In 2024 and 2025, we saw the FDA and European approval of transcatheter tricuspid devices (like the TriClip and Evoque systems).

The Impact: In your 2026 clinics, you will see patients with massive leg swelling and liver congestion from "Torrential Tricuspid Regurgitation." Previously, we just gave them diuretics. Now, you will be assessing them for "Edge-to-Edge Repair" (TEER).

New Skill: You need to learn the Transgastric Views on TO (Transoesophageal Echo) to visualise the tricuspid leaflets properly. It is technically harder than the mitral valve.

4.2 AI-Assisted Echocardiography

We are not replacing sonographers, but we are augmenting them.

Automated Strain Imaging: Global Longitudinal Strain (GLS) is now a standard button press. It detects LV dysfunction before the Ejection Fraction (EF) drops. In cardio-oncology (chemo patients), this is vital.

Auto-Doppler: The machine now automatically traces the spectral Doppler envelopes to calculate gradients. Your job is to ensure the machine hasn't tracked a ghost signal (artefact).

4.3 The "Asymptomatic" TAVI

The EARLY TAVR trial results have changed our waiting lists. We used to wait for symptoms (breathlessness/chest pain) before replacing an aortic valve. We now know that "watchful waiting" often leads to irreversible damage.

2026 Practice: If you see a patient with critical AS (Velocity > 4.5 m/s) who claims to be "asymptomatic," we now stress test them or look for subtle markers (like BNP elevation or GLS drop) to justify early intervention.

2. Subtopic 5.3: Advanced Imaging Modalities

In the modern NHS, the "Triple Assessment" for chest pain often relies heavily on advanced imaging. The days of relying solely on exercise tolerance testing (ETT) for diagnosis are largely behind us. We now rely on anatomical precision (CT), tissue characterization (MRI), and metabolic function (Nuclear).

2.1 Cardiac Computed Tomography (CCT)

Cardiac CT has arguably seen the most explosive growth of any modality in the last decade. By 2026, it has cemented itself as the first-line investigation for stable chest pain in patients with low-to-moderate clinical likelihood of coronary artery disease (CAD), as per the paradigm shift in the 2024 ESC Guidelines for Chronic Coronary Syndromes.

The Core Competency: Reporting Under Supervision The curriculum is specific here: you must be able to report CT coronary angiograms (CTCA) under direct supervision. This means sitting at the workstation, manipulating the multi-planar reconstructions (MPR), and identifying the three main coronary arteries.

Anatomy: You need to identify the Left Main Stem (LMS), Left Anterior Descending (LAD), Circumflex (Cx), and Right Coronary Artery (RCA). You must also recognize dominance (usually right-dominant) and anomalies.

The "Soft" Plaque vs. Calcified Plaque: CT is excellent at spotting calcification (the "calcium score"). However, in 2026, we are more interested in non-calcified or "soft" plaque, which is the substrate for acute coronary syndromes. A patient might have a calcium score of zero but still have a dangerous soft plaque in the proximal LAD.

Example: Consider a 45-year-old male smoker presenting with atypical chest pain. His EKG is normal. A decade ago, he might have had an exercise treadmill test. Today, you order a CTCA. The scan reveals a Calcium Score of 0, but the contrast-enhanced images show a tight, non-calcified lesion in the mid-LAD. This "soft" plaque is high-risk. Because you ordered the CT, you caught a lesion that a stress test might have missed if the ischemia wasn't severe enough to cause EKG changes yet.

FFR-CT: The 2026 Standard One of the biggest leaps we've seen is the integration of FFR-CT (Fractional Flow Reserve derived from CT). Historically, CT was criticized for over-calling stenosis—it often made moderate disease look severe. FFR-CT uses computational fluid dynamics to virtually simulate pressure wires.

If a lesion looks like 50-70% stenosis on CT, we no longer just send them for an angiogram. We run the FFR-CT analysis.

If the value is >0.80, it is non-ischemic. The patient needs statins, not stents.

If the value is <0.75, it is likely ischemia-causing. The patient proceeds to the cath lab.

Risks and Limitations As a trainee, you must respect the radiation dose, although modern scanners with "flash" protocols have reduced this to sub-millisievert levels (less than a year of background radiation). The bigger limitation is heart rate. To "freeze" the heart, the rate needs to be below 60-65 bpm.

Practical Tip: You will often be the one prescribing oral or IV beta-blockers (like Metoprolol) in the scanner waiting room. You must screen for asthma and heart block before doing this.

2.2 Cardiac Magnetic Resonance (CMR)

If CT is the camera that looks at the pipes, MRI is the camera that looks at the walls. It is the gold standard for tissue characterization. It uses no radiation, relying instead on magnetic fields and radio waves.

The "Working Knowledge" Required You don't need to know the physics of "k-space," but you must know what "Late Gadolinium Enhancement" (LGE) implies. Gadolinium is an extracellular contrast agent. In healthy heart muscle, the cells are tightly packed, and gadolinium washes out quickly. In scarred or fibrotic heart muscle, the space between cells is expanded, and gadolinium gets "stuck" or washes out slowly. This shows up as bright white on the scan.

Differentiation of Cardiomyopathy This is the superpower of CMR. It can distinguish why a heart is weak.

Ischemic Cardiomyopathy: The scarring (LGE) starts from the inside (sub-endocardial) and moves outward. This follows a vascular territory (e.g., the LAD territory).

Non-Ischemic Dilated Cardiomyopathy (DCM): The scarring is often in the mid-wall of the septum (a "mid-wall stripe").

Myocarditis: The scarring is often on the outside (sub-epicardial) and patchy.

Example: You admit a 30-year-old female with chest pain, raised troponins, but clean coronary arteries on the angiogram. The working diagnosis is "MINOCA" (Myocardial Infarction with Non-Obstructive Coronary Arteries). What do you do? You order a CMR. The scan shows patchy sub-epicardial enhancement in the lateral wall. This confirms acute myocarditis, likely viral. This changes the management completely—she doesn't need antiplatelets; she needs rest and supportive care.

Stress Perfusion CMR For detecting ischemia, Stress CMR is a robust alternative to nuclear scans or stress echo. We use Adenosine to dilate the blood vessels. Healthy vessels dilate, and blood flow increases. Diseased vessels cannot dilate further. The MRI tracks the "first pass" of contrast. Dark areas during stress indicate ischemia.

2.3 Nuclear Cardiology

Nuclear cardiology often feels like the "older sibling" to the flashy CT and MRI, but it remains a workhorse, particularly for specific questions regarding viability and infiltration.

SPECT (Single Photon Emission Computed Tomography) This is the traditional "myoview." It is excellent for patients who cannot do an MRI (e.g., those with old pacemakers or severe claustrophobia). However, it carries a radiation burden.

Indication: Assessing ischemia in a patient with known heavy calcification (where CT fails) or metallic devices (where MRI fails).

PET (Positron Emission Tomography) PET is the gold standard for Viability.

The Question: "This patient has an occluded LAD and an ejection fraction of 25%. If we bypass the LAD, will the muscle wake up?"

The Mismatch: We look for "Perfusion-Metabolism Mismatch." We inject FDG (glucose). If the heart muscle takes up glucose (it is alive/eating) but has poor blood flow (perfusion defect), the muscle is hibernating. Revascularization will help. If there is no glucose uptake, it is scar tissue. Revascularization is futile.

Amyloidosis: The Modern Renaissance The most vital "2026 update" for a trainee in nuclear cardiology is Transthyretin Amyloidosis (ATTR).

We use bone scintigraphy tracers (like DPD or PYP).

Strangely, these bone tracers stick avidly to the heart if it is infiltrated with TTR amyloid.

The "Perugini Grade": If the heart takes up more tracer than the ribs (Grade 2 or 3), and blood tests rule out light-chain (AL) amyloid, you can diagnose Cardiac Amyloidosis without a biopsy.

Why it matters: In 2026, we have drugs like Tafamidis and gene silencers that treat this. Diagnosing it early is no longer academic; it saves lives.

Example: An 80-year-old man has "heart failure with preserved ejection fraction" (HFpEF). His echo shows thick walls. You suspect amyloid. You order a DPD bone scan. The heart lights up black on the scan (Grade 3 uptake). You have just diagnosed ATTR cardiomyopathy. You refer him to the specialist service for stabilizing therapy.

3. Subtopic 5.4: Aortopathy and Inherited Structural Conditions

This section of the curriculum deals with the "silent killers." Aortopathies are diseases of the aorta that predispose it to dilation and dissection. Unlike coronary disease, which hurts (angina), the aorta often grows silently until it tears.

3.1 The Spectrum of Aortopathy

You must be familiar with the "Syndromic" and "Non-Syndromic" causes.

Syndromic Aortopathies:

Marfan Syndrome (FBN1 mutation): The classic connective tissue disorder. Patients are tall, have long fingers (arachnodactyly), and lens dislocation (ectopia lentis). The danger zone is the Aortic Root (Sinus of Valsalva).

Loeys-Dietz Syndrome (TGFBR1/2): More aggressive than Marfan. The aorta can dissect at smaller diameters. Key features include a bifid uvula and hypertelorism (wide-set eyes).

Vascular Ehlers-Danlos (COL3A1): The most terrifying variant. The tissue is friable (like wet tissue paper). Surgery is extremely difficult. We avoid invasive catheters if possible because the arteries can tear easily.

Non-Syndromic / Bicuspid Aortopathy: Bicuspid Aortic Valve (BAV) is the most common congenital heart defect (1-2% of the population). Roughly 50% of BAV patients will develop aortic dilation.

The Association: BAV is not just a valve problem; it is an aortopathy. The aorta can dilate even if the valve is functioning well.

3.2 Management: Surveillance vs. Surgery

The core skill here is Risk Stratification. When do we operate? In the UK, we follow the ESC Guidelines and the Aortic Dissection Detection Risk Score.

Surveillance: Patients with known dilation need serial imaging. Echo is good, but CT or MRI is required to see the whole arch and descending aorta. "Working knowledge" means knowing that measurements must be taken essentially perpendicular to the flow of blood (the "double oblique" technique).

The Thresholds (General Rule of Thumb for 2026):

5.5 cm: Surgery recommended for the general population (degenerative aneurysm).

5.0 cm: Surgery recommended for Bicuspid Valve patients with risk factors (or Marfan).

4.5 cm: Surgery recommended for Marfan patients with risk factors (family history of dissection) or Loeys-Dietz.

Growth Rate: Rapid growth (>3-5mm per year) triggers surgery regardless of absolute size.

Example: You see a 25-year-old man in the clinic. He is 6'6" with a concave chest. He has never seen a doctor. You suspect Marfan. His echo shows an aortic root of 4.8 cm. This is a critical finding. You do not just book a follow-up in a year. You refer him to the "Aorta MDT" (Multidisciplinary Team). He likely needs prophylactic "Valve-Sparing Root Replacement" (David Procedure) to prevent a dissection that could kill him.

3.3 Acute Aortic Syndromes

You must recognize the presentation. It is not always "tearing back pain."

Type A Dissection: Involves the ascending aorta. Surgical Emergency. Mortality increases 1-2% per hour.

Action: Control BP (IV Labetalol, target systolic <120 mmHg) and call the surgeons immediately.

Type B Dissection: Involves the descending aorta only. Medical Management (usually).

Action: Strict BP control. We only operate (TEVAR - Thoracic Endovascular Aortic Repair) if there are complications like malperfusion (gut ischemia, cold leg) or rupture.

3.4 Family Screening and ICC Services

The curriculum emphasizes that your job doesn't end with the patient. "The patient is the family; the family is the patient."

If you find a Bicuspid Valve or a unexplained thoracic aneurysm in a young person, you must recommend screening for first-degree relatives (parents, siblings, children).

Inherited Cardiac Conditions (ICC) Clinic: These are specialized clinics in the UK. Your role as a core trainee is to identify the "proband" (the first affected family member) and refer them to the ICC service for genetic counselling and cascade testing.

Example: A 50-year-old man presents with a Type A dissection. He survives surgery. His history reveals his father died suddenly at 45. This suggests Familial Thoracic Aortic Aneurysm and Dissection (FTAAD). You must ensure his children are screened. If they carry the ACTA2 gene mutation, they are at risk and need monitoring from childhood.

3.5 Pregnancy and Structural Heart Disease

This is a "Red Flag" area in the curriculum. Pregnancy places a massive haemodynamic burden on the cardiovascular system (50% increase in blood volume).

Pre-Conceptual Counselling:

Women with Marfan syndrome and an aortic root >4.0 - 4.5 cm are at extremely high risk of dissection during pregnancy or the postpartum period.

They should be counselled against pregnancy until the aorta is repaired.

If they are already pregnant, they need management in a tertiary center with cardiac obstetrics.

WHO Classification of Maternal Risk:

WHO IV (Pregnancy Contraindicated): Severe symptomatic aortic stenosis, Marfan with aorta >4.5cm, severe coarctation.

Management: Regular echo surveillance during pregnancy. Strict BP control. Beta-blockers are often continued (labetalol or bisoprolol) despite small risks of fetal growth restriction, because the risk to the mother is life-threatening.

Example: A 28-year-old woman with known Bicuspid Aortic Valve and a 4.2cm aorta wants to get pregnant. She asks you if it is safe.

Your Answer: It is not "zero risk." She falls into WHO Class II-III. The risk of dissection is elevated but manageable. She will need an echo every trimester. She needs to deliver in a hospital with cardiothoracic surgery on site, just in case. You must refer her to the "Maternal Cardiology" joint clinic.

Core Theme: Electrophysiology and Devices

1. Introduction to the Module

Welcome to the Core Capabilities in Practice (CiP) module on Electrophysiology. In the rapidly evolving landscape of cardiology, the management of heart rhythm disorders has shifted from a purely reactive discipline to one driven by precision medicine, advanced technology, and integrated care pathways.

This course material is designed for the modern cardiology trainee. It moves beyond the dry recitation of guidelines and delves into the art of arrhythmia management—understanding the physiological storms that rage within the unwell patient and the nuanced, long-term strategies required for chronic care. We will explore the 2026 standards of care, incorporating the latest directives from the European Society of Cardiology (ESC 2024/25) and the Resuscitation Council UK (2025 updates).

This module is divided into two critical sections: the high-stakes management of the acutely unwell patient (6.1) and the longitudinal, complex management of chronic arrhythmias (6.2).

2. Acute Arrhythmia Management (6.1)

The management of the acutely unwell patient with arrhythmia is perhaps the most adrenaline-charged aspect of cardiology. It requires a cool head, rapid decision-making, and a mastery of physiology. We are not just treating an ECG trace; we are stabilizing a failing hemodynamic system.

The "Unwell" Patient: A Physiological Crisis

When a patient presents with acute arrhythmia, the immediate priority is not diagnosis, but stability. The 2025 Resuscitation Council UK guidelines re-emphasize the "ABCDE" approach, but with a nuanced appreciation for the reversible causes specific to electrophysiology.

The term "unwell" in this context refers to the presence of adverse features: shock (hypotension, pallor, sweating), syncope, myocardial ischaemia, or severe heart failure. In these scenarios, the luxury of time—and often the utility of drugs—is removed. Electricity (DC cardioversion) becomes the primary therapeutic agent.

Electrical Storm: The Sympathetic Surge

Electrical Storm (ES) is defined as three or more distinct episodes of sustained ventricular arrhythmia within a 24-hour period. It is a medical emergency that carries a high mortality rate if not aggressively managed. The 2025 consensus views ES not just as an electrical failure, but as a sympathetic crisis. The patient's anxiety and pain drive a catecholamine surge, which in turn fuels further arrhythmia, creating a vicious cycle.

Sympathetic Blockade: This is the cornerstone of modern management. We are moving away from purely relying on Amiodarone. The use of non-selective beta-blockers, such as Propranolol, is increasingly favoured (unless contraindicated by severe heart failure) because they block both beta-1 and beta-2 receptors, effectively dampening the adrenergic storm.

Deep Sedation: Never underestimate the power of sedation. Intubation and ventilation are not just for airway protection here; they are anti-arrhythmic interventions. By removing the patient's conscious drive and sympathetic outflow, we often terminate the storm when drugs fail.

2026 Interventional Perspective: If the storm persists despite maximal medical therapy (amiodarone, lidocaine, beta-blockade), the patient requires urgent transfer to a tertiary centre. The 2025 guidelines support early consideration of catheter ablation or neuraxial modulation (like stellate ganglion block) to mechanically interrupt the circuit. In extremis, ECMO (Extracorporeal Membrane Oxygenation) serves as a bridge to ablation.

Wide-Complex Tachycardia (WCT): Diagnostic Precision

One of the most intimidating presentations on the acute take is the Wide-Complex Tachycardia. The golden rule remains: Treat as Ventricular Tachycardia (VT) until proven otherwise.

Misidentifying VT as SVT with aberrancy can be fatal. If you administer Verapamil to a patient in VT, you may precipitate cardiac arrest by causing vasodilation in a heart that is relying on vasoconstriction to maintain pressure.

The 2026 Pharmacological Shift: While Amiodarone remains a standard, recent data (including the PROCAMIO trial insights) suggests Procainamide (where available) may offer better termination rates with fewer adverse cardiac events for stable VT, though its availability in the UK remains variable.

DC Cardioversion: Trainees must be independent in this skill. It is not merely about pressing a button; it involves safe sedation, synchronization to the R-wave to avoid "R-on-T" phenomena (which can trigger V-Fib), and airway management.

Severe Bradycardia and Pacing Skills

Bradycardia management has been refined in the Resus Council UK 2025 guidelines. The dosing of Atropine (500mcg–1mg IV) remains the first line for vagally mediated blocks. However, for high-grade AV block (Mobitz II or Complete Heart Block), particularly in the context of anterior MI, drugs are often unreliable.

Temporary Pacing (Level 3/4 Competence): Inserting a temporary pacing wire is a critical "rescue skill" for the medical registrar. In an era where transcutaneous (pad) pacing is widely available, the art of inserting a transvenous wire is sometimes neglected, yet it is essential for patients who cannot tolerate the pain of external pacing or who require pacing for days rather than hours.

Safety First: The procedure is now almost exclusively performed under ultrasound guidance/fluoroscopy to minimize the risk of pneumothorax and vascular injury.

The "Bridge": Remember, temporary pacing is a bridge—to recovery (e.g., drug toxicity resolution), to a permanent pacemaker, or to decision-making.

3. Chronic Arrhythmia and Anticoagulation (6.2)

Moving from the acute to the chronic, we encounter the bread and butter of cardiology: Atrial Fibrillation (AF). By 2026, the management of AF has been revolutionized by new ablation technologies and a holistic care pathway.
The AF-CARE Pathway (ESC 2024/25)

We no longer simply "rate control and anticoagulate." The European Society of Cardiology has codified the AF-CARE pathway, which trainees must internalize:

[C] Comorbidity & Risk Factor Management: AF is often a symptom of systemic ill health. Managing hypertension, obesity (aiming for >10% weight loss), sleep apnoea, and alcohol reduction is as "anti-arrhythmic" as any drug.

[A] Avoid Stroke & Thromboembolism: This is the non-negotiable safety step.

[R] Reduce Symptoms: Through rate or rhythm control.

[E] Evaluate & Reassess: AF is progressive; management must be dynamic.

Stroke Prevention: The New Precision

Risk stratification has evolved. We use the CHA2DS2-VA score (a refinement of CHA2DS2-VASc), which removes "female sex" as an independent risk factor, acknowledging that women are only at higher risk if they have other comorbidities.

Anticoagulation: DOACs (Direct Oral Anticoagulants)—Apixaban, Edoxaban, Rivaroxaban, Dabigatran—are the standard of care. Warfarin is now relegated to specific niches: mechanical heart valves and Antiphospholipid Syndrome.

Complex Scenarios:

The Frail/Elderly: Age is the strongest driver of stroke risk. We do not withhold anticoagulation solely due to fall risk. The benefit of stroke prevention almost always outweighs the risk of a bleed from a fall.

Renal Impairment: This is a delicate balance. While some DOACs are contraindicated in severe failure (eGFR

<15), 2026 practice often sees close collaboration with nephrology, sometimes utilizing reduced-dose regimens or Warfarin with tight control, though the evidence base in dialysis patients remains contentious.

LAA Occlusion: For patients who absolutely cannot tolerate anticoagulation (e.g., recurrent severe GI bleeds), Left Atrial Appendage occlusion is a vital structural alternative.

Rhythm Control: The Rise of Pulsed Field Ablation (PFA)

Perhaps the most exciting development in the 2025/2026 curriculum is the widespread adoption of Pulsed Field Ablation (PFA).

For decades, we burned (Radiofrequency) or froze (Cryo) the heart to isolate pulmonary veins. These thermal energies carried collateral risks—damaging the oesophagus or phrenic nerve. PFA uses high-voltage, microsecond electrical pulses to create pores in the cell membranes (electroporation).

Tissue Selectivity: The magic of PFA is that cardiomyocytes have a specific threshold for this energy. We can ablate the arrhythmia substrate while sparing the oesophagus, nerves, and blood vessels, which are resistant to the same energy levels.

NICE IPG806 (July 2025): The UK's National Institute for Health and Care Excellence has recognized PFA, leading to its rapid rollout across NHS trusts. Trainees today must understand that "early rhythm control" (ablation as a first-line therapy) is now superior to drug therapy for maintaining sinus rhythm and improving quality of life, especially in heart failure patients.

1.1 The Evolution of Patient Selection

The decision to implant a device is one of the most consequential moments in a patient's care. In 2026, the binary choice between "pacemaker" and "defibrillator" has evolved into a nuanced selection of physiological pacing modalities.

Pacemakers (Bradycardia Management): The foundational indication remains symptomatic bradycardia (Sick Sinus Syndrome or AV block). However, the method of pacing has changed.

Historical Context: Historically, we paced the Right Ventricular (RV) apex. We now know this causes dyssynchrony—an electrical "wobble" that can weaken the heart over time.

2026 Standard: The trainee must now consider Conduction System Pacing (CSP) as a frontline option. Instead of burying a lead in the muscle, we screw the lead directly into the heart's natural wiring (the His Bundle or the Left Bundle Branch Area). This restores a narrow, natural heartbeat.

Selection Criteria: If a patient is expected to require >40% ventricular pacing, CSP or Cardiac Resynchronization Therapy (CRT) is preferred over standard RV pacing to prevent pacing-induced cardiomyopathy.

ICDs (Sudden Death Prevention): Implantable Cardioverter Defibrillators (ICDs) act as paramedics in the chest.

Primary Prevention: We implant these in patients who have not had an arrest but are at high risk (e.g., Ischaemic cardiomyopathy with LVEF <30-35% despite optimal medical therapy).

Secondary Prevention: Used for survivors of cardiac arrest or sustained Ventricular Tachycardia (VT).

The Subcutaneous ICD (S-ICD): By 2026, the S-ICD (which sits under the skin, not in the heart) is the preferred choice for younger patients without pacing needs. It eliminates the risk of lead infection entering the bloodstream.

Cardiac Resynchronization Therapy (CRT): CRT is "tuning" the engine. It is indicated for heart failure patients with a wide QRS complex (typically Left Bundle Branch Block, LBBB).

The Mechanism: By pacing both the left and right ventricles, we resynchronize the contraction.

The "Non-Responder" Problem: Not everyone improves with CRT. In 2026, we increasingly use Left Bundle Branch Area Pacing (LBBAP) as an alternative to traditional biventricular CRT, especially for patients who have difficult anatomy or have failed conventional CRT.

1.2 Core Trainee Competencies: Interrogation and Programming

While implantation is a consultant-level skill, the Core Trainee is the first line of defense on the wards. You must be "device literate." This does not mean you need to know how to install the wiring, but you must know how to check the fuse box.

The Basic Interrogation (The "Check"): When you place a programmer head on a patient's chest, you are looking for three "vital signs" of the device:

Battery Status: Is it reaching "ERI" (Elective Replacement Indicator)? If so, an elective generator change is needed. If it hits "EOS" (End of Service), it is an emergency.

Lead Impedance: Think of this as the resistance in the wire.

Sudden Drop (<200 ohms): Suggests an insulation break (short circuit).

Sudden Rise (>2000 ohms): Suggests a lead fracture (broken wire).

Sensing and Thresholds:

Sensing: Can the device "see" the patient's own heartbeat? (measured in millivolts).

Threshold: How much energy does it take to capture the heart? (measured in volts).

Emergency Programming: There are two scenarios where a trainee must act instantly:

Inappropriate Shocks: If a patient is awake and getting shocked repeatedly (e.g., due to a lead fracture or rapid Atrial Fibrillation being misread as VT), you must apply a magnet. In 2026, clinical magnets are standard on all crash trolleys. Placing a magnet over an ICD suspends detection—it blinds the device so it stops shocking, but it does not stop pacing.

Peri-operative Management: Before surgery using diathermy (electrocautery), a pacemaker might interpret the electrical interference as a heart rhythm and inhibit pacing (stop working). The trainee must program the device to an "asynchronous" mode (e.g., VOO or DOO), forcing it to pace at a fixed rate regardless of interference.

1.3 Complications: Recognition and Management

Devices are foreign bodies; the body sometimes rejects them, or mechanics fail.

Infection (The Red Flag): Never ignore a red, angry generator pocket.

Rule of Thumb: If there is pus, erosion, or systemic sepsis with a device, the entire system (box and leads) must be extracted. Antibiotics alone are a holding measure, not a cure.

Lead Displacement: Common in the first 6 weeks.

Scenario: A patient with a new pacemaker faints. An X-ray shows the lead tip has pulled back from the ventricle ("Twiddler's Syndrome" or poor fixation). This requires urgent re-operation.

Pneumothorax: A collapsed lung during implantation. Small ones (<2cm) observed; large ones require a chest drain.

Section 2: Inherited Arrhythmia Syndromes (ICC) – Subtopic 6.4

2.1 The Channelopathies: Electrical Storms in Normal Hearts

Inherited Cardiac Conditions (ICCs) are the silent killers of the young. These patients have structurally normal hearts (normal echo) but genetically faulty ion channels.

Long QT Syndrome (LQTS):

The Pathology: A delay in repolarization (recharging) of the heart, predisposing to Torsades de Pointes.

Triggers:

LQT1: Triggered by exercise (typically swimming).

LQT2: Triggered by auditory shock (alarm clocks, doorbells).

LQT3: Occurs during sleep/rest.

Management: Beta-blockers (specifically Nadolol or Propranolol) are the mainstay. High-risk patients may need an ICD or Left Cardiac Sympathetic Denervation (cutting the nerve supply to calm the heart).

Brugada Syndrome:

The Look: A "coved" ST-segment elevation in leads V1-V2.

The Danger: Sudden death during sleep or fever.

2026 Management Update: We are more conservative with ICDs in asymptomatic Brugada than we were a decade ago. Aggressive fever management and avoidance of specific drugs are the first line.

Catecholaminergic Polymorphic VT (CPVT):

The Scenario: A child faints during sports or emotional stress. The ECG is normal at rest.

The Test: An exercise tolerance test reveals bidirectional VT.

The Treatment: High-dose beta-blockers and Flecainide. This is one of the most lethal conditions if untreated.

2.2 Sudden Arrhythmic Death Syndrome (SADS)

When a young person (<40) dies suddenly and the autopsy is normal, it is labeled SADS. This is a "sentinel event" for the family.

The Role of the Trainee: You are not just treating a patient; you are treating a pedigree. If you identify a SADS case, you must refer the first-degree relatives (parents, siblings, children) for screening.

The Screen: ECG, Echocardiogram, and Exercise Test.

The "Molecular Autopsy": In 2026, post-mortem genetic testing of the deceased is standard. If a mutation is found, we can test the relatives for that specific gene ("cascade screening"), saving them from years of uncertainty.

2.3 Psychosocial and Socioeconomic Impact

A diagnosis of an inherited arrhythmia carries a heavy burden. It acts as a "biological criminal record" that can limit freedom.

Driving (DVLA/RSA Guidelines 2025/2026): Driving regulations are strict because a faint at the wheel is fatal.

Group 1 (Car):

Symptomatic (Syncope): Must stop driving. Can restart after symptoms are controlled for 4 weeks (or 6 months depending on severity).

ICD Implant: If implanted for secondary prevention (after an arrest), the ban is 6 months. If the device delivers a shock, the clock resets.

Group 2 (HGV/Bus):

Usually a permanent bar. A diagnosis of Brugada or Long QT with a history of syncope often disqualifies a patient from holding a vocational license. This leads to immediate job loss, requiring sensitive counseling.

Lifestyle & Employment:

The "Cotton Wool" Kid: Parents of children with ICCs often restrict them from all play. The trainee must encourage "safe" activity. We no longer ban all sports—guidelines now allow recreational sport for most stable patients, promoting mental health.

Insurance: Patients may struggle to get life insurance or travel cover. Signposting to specialist advocacy groups (like Cardiomyopathy UK or SADS UK) is a clinical duty.

Core Theme: Adult Congenital Heart Disease (ACHD)

Part 1: Recognition and Initial Management (Subtopic 7.1)

In the UK, the majority of complex CHD is diagnosed antenatally or in infancy. However, "simple" shunts and obstructive lesions often slip through the net, only to surface when the physiological reserves of adulthood begin to fade.

1. The Hidden Shunts: Atrial Septal Defect (ASD)

The ASD is the chameleon of cardiology. It is the most common congenital heart defect found in adults who were previously undiagnosed.

Anatomy & Pathophysiology: Imagine a hole in the septum separating the left and right atria. Because left atrial pressure is marginally higher than the right, oxygenated blood shunts left-to-right. This doesn't cause cyanosis (blue skin) initially. Instead, it creates a volume overload. The right ventricle (RV) and pulmonary arteries are flooded with extra blood, leading to gradual dilatation.
Shutterstock

The "2026" Clinical Picture: You likely won't see a "sick" patient. You will see a 45-year-old who mentions they used to run 5k but now get tired after 2k.

The Clues: A fixed split second heart sound (due to delayed pulmonary valve closure from extra volume) is the hallmark, but hard to hear. More commonly, they present with new-onset Atrial Fibrillation (AF) or a Right Bundle

Branch Block (RBBB) on an ECG found during a routine check-up.

The Trap: Treating the AF without looking for the cause. If you see unexplained RV dilatation on an echo, hunt for the ASD.

Initial Management: If you suspect an ASD, do not rush to refer immediately without data.

Confirm: Transthoracic Echo (TTE) is the first line. If the windows are poor, a Transoesophageal Echo (TOE) or Cardiac MRI is the gold standard in 2026.

Manage: If they are in heart failure, diuretics may be needed. If in AF, rate control and anticoagulation are critical—these patients are at high risk of paradoxical emboli (clots crossing the hole and causing a stroke).

2. The Loud Rumble: Ventricular Septal Defect (VSD)

Unlike the subtle ASD, a VSD is often noisy.

Anatomy: A hole between the ventricles.

Pathophysiology: The pressure difference between the Left Ventricle (LV) and Right Ventricle (RV) is massive (e.g., 120mmHg vs 25mmHg). This drives a high-velocity jet of blood into the RV. Paradoxically, smaller holes make louder murmurs because of the higher turbulence.

The "Eisenmenger" Fear: If a large VSD is left untreated for decades, the high pressure damages the lungs' blood vessels permanently (Pulmonary Vascular Disease). Eventually, the pressure in the lungs exceeds the body's pressure, and the shunt reverses (right-to-left). The patient turns blue (cyanotic). This is inoperable.

Real-World Example: A patient in their 30s with clubbed fingers and oxygen saturation of 85% likely has Eisenmenger physiology. Do not give them oxygen; it won't help the shunt. Refer to a tertiary centre immediately.

3. The Silent Hypertension: Coarctation of the Aorta

This is a narrowing of the aorta, usually just after the arch. Think of it like a kink in a garden hose.

The Presentation: The pressure builds up before the kink (head and arms) and drops after the kink (legs).

Scenario: You see a 28-year-old male with resistant hypertension (180/100 mmHg). He is on three drugs, and nothing is working.

The Test: Feel the pulses. His radial (wrist) pulse will be bounding, but his femoral (groin) pulse will be weak or delayed. This is "radio-femoral delay."
Shutterstock

Initial Management:

BP Control: Aggressive blood pressure control is vital to prevent a stroke or aortic dissection. Beta-blockers are often used.

Imaging: A CT Aorta or MRI is required to visualize the narrowing.

Referral: They will likely need a stent or surgery.

Part 2: The Transition from Paediatric Services (Subtopic 7.2)

This is arguably the most complex part of the curriculum because it deals with psychology, not just physiology. "Transition" is not a single event; it is a process that occurs between ages 14 and 18+.

1. The Vulnerable Gap

Between the ages of 16 and 19, patients are most likely to be "lost to follow-up." They leave the protective wing of their parents and the paediatric team but feel too intimidated or "well" to attend an adult clinic.

The Risk: A young adult with a repaired heart often feels "cured." They stop taking meds, start smoking, or ignore symptoms.

Your Role: You are not just a doctor here; you are a negotiator. You must ensure they understand that "repaired" does not mean "fixed."

2. Psychosocial Challenges

Adolescence is hard enough. Add a zipper scar down your chest, and it becomes a minefield.

Body Image: Young patients may avoid swimming or intimacy due to surgical scars.

Risk-Taking: Adolescents with ACHD often engage in more risk-taking behaviours (alcohol, drugs) than their peers as a form of rebellion against their "fragile" label.

Vocational Advice: They need honest conversations about careers. A patient on warfarin cannot be a rugby player; a patient with a pacemaker might face restrictions in the military or electrical engineering.

3. The "Ready Steady Go" Approach

In the UK (as of the 2025/2026 guidelines), transition clinics use a structured empowerment model:

Ready (Age 14-15): The doctor starts addressing the patient, not the parents. "Do you know the name of your heart condition?"

Steady (Age 16-17): The patient is seen alone for part of the consultation. They learn about their medications and side effects.

Go (Age 18+): Transfer to the ACHD centre. They should confidently know when to seek help and how to navigate the NHS.

Part 3: Long-Term Sequelae of Repairs

The curriculum requires you to manage patients who had surgery decades ago. The classic example is Tetralogy of Fallot (ToF).

1. Tetralogy of Fallot: Repaired, but at a Cost

ToF is the most common cyanotic defect repaired in childhood. It involves four defects (VSD, Pulmonary Stenosis, Overriding Aorta, RV Hypertrophy). Surgeons patch the VSD and widen the pulmonary valve.

The Consequence: Widening the pulmonary valve often leaves it "incompetent." It leaks.

Pulmonary Regurgitation (PR): Over 20–30 years, severe PR causes the Right Ventricle to dilate and fail.

The Danger Zone: As the RV stretches, it becomes electrically unstable. This creates a substrate for Ventricular Tachycardia (VT). Sudden cardiac death is the leading cause of mortality in adult ToF patients.

Management in 2026:

Surveillance: These patients need annual MRI scans to measure RV volume.

Intervention: We no longer wait for symptoms. If the RV gets too big (indexed volume >150ml/m^2), we replace the valve (Pulmonary Valve Replacement - PVR), often via a catheter (percutaneous) rather than open-heart surgery.

2. Palliated Physiology: The Fontan Circulation

Some hearts cannot be repaired (e.g., those born with only one ventricle). Instead, they are "palliated." The Fontan procedure reroutes all the blue blood from the body directly to the lungs, bypassing the heart entirely. The single ventricle then pumps only red blood to the body.

The Reality: Blood flows to the lungs passively, without a pump. This relies entirely on low lung pressures.

The Failing Fontan: In adulthood, these patients essentially live in a state of chronic venous congestion.

Protein-Losing Enteropathy: The gut swells, and they lose protein in stool.

Plastic Bronchitis: They cough up cast-like moulds of their airways.

Liver Cirrhosis: The high venous pressure stiffens the liver ("Fontan Liver").

Your Role: Any deterioration in a Fontan patient (swelling, arrhythmia, fatigue) is a red flag. They tolerate arrhythmias very poorly. A simple AF can be fatal because they lose the "kick" needed to push blood through the lungs.

Part 1: Pregnancy in ACHD (Subtopic 7.3)

1.1 The Physiological "Stress Test" of Pregnancy

To counsel a patient effectively, you must first respect the sheer magnitude of the hemodynamic burden pregnancy places on the body. We often tell patients that pregnancy is like running a marathon that lasts nine months, but physiologically, it is more like a sustained stress test.

By the second trimester (around 24 weeks), the maternal body undergoes profound changes:

Plasma Volume Expansion: The blood volume increases by nearly 50%. Imagine the heart, which may already be compromised by congenital defects, suddenly needing to handle half again as much fluid.

Drop in Systemic Vascular Resistance (SVR): The placenta is essentially a low-resistance shunt. It demands blood flow, causing the mother's blood vessels to dilate. This drops the blood pressure.

Heart Rate Increase: To maintain pressure despite the dilated vessels, the heart rate rises by 10–20 beats per minute.

The "Cliff Edge" for ACHD Patients For a normal heart, these changes are manageable. For an ACHD heart, they can be catastrophic.

Example: Consider a patient with severe aortic stenosis. Her heart struggles to pump blood out through a narrowed valve. When pregnancy demands a 50% increase in output, the heart simply cannot keep up. The result can be sudden pulmonary edema (fluid in the lungs).

Example: Consider a patient with Eisenmenger syndrome (severe pulmonary hypertension). Her life depends on high systemic pressure to prevent right-to-left shunting (blue blood mixing with red). When pregnancy drops her SVR (blood pressure), blue blood floods her system, causing life-threatening cyanosis for both mother and baby.

1.2 Pre-Pregnancy Counselling: The "Taboo" Conversation

In 2026, the standard of care is proactive, not reactive. We do not wait for a patient to become pregnant to discuss risks. The conversation begins at age 12 or 13. This is known as "reproductive counseling."

The mWHO Classification (Modified World Health Organization) We use the mWHO risk score to give patients a realistic picture of their safety. It is the gold standard in the UK curriculum.

mWHO I (Low Risk): Risks are similar to the general population.

Examples: Successfully repaired ASD, VSD, or PDA with no residual issues.

mWHO II (Moderate Risk): A small increase in maternal mortality or morbidity.

Examples: Unoperated ASD, Repaired Tetralogy of Fallot without major valve leaks.

mWHO III (High Risk): Significant risk. Pregnancy requires a "Pregnancy Heart Team" and intense monitoring.

Examples: Mechanical valves, Systemic Right Ventricle (like in Transposition of the Great Arteries), Fontan circulation.

mWHO IV (Prohibitive Risk): Pregnancy is contraindicated because the risk of death is too high.

Examples: Pulmonary Arterial Hypertension (PAH), severe ventricular dysfunction (LVEF <30%), severe mitral stenosis.

Crucial Note for Trainees: If a patient falls into mWHO IV, your duty is to gently but clearly advise against pregnancy. However, if she chooses to proceed (as is her human right), we do not abandon her. We assemble the multidisciplinary team to mitigate risk as much as possible.

1.3 Contraception: Navigating the Estrogen Minefield

Trainees often overlook contraception, yet it is a lethal blind spot. A woman with a mechanical heart valve or Fontan circulation has a high risk of thrombosis (clots).

The Danger of Estrogen: Combined oral contraceptives (the "Pill") containing estrogen are pro-thrombotic. They make blood sticky. Giving the Pill to a woman with a mechanical valve is akin to lighting a match near gasoline; the risk of valve thrombosis and stroke is unacceptable.

The Safe Alternatives:

Progesterone-only methods: The "Mini-pill," the implant (Nexplanon), or the coil (Mirena). These do not increase clot risk significantly.

Intrauterine Devices (IUDs): Highly effective. However, insertion can cause a "vasovagal" reaction (slowing of the heart), which can be dangerous in Fontan patients. It should be done in a hospital setting, not a GP surgery, for high-risk ACHD patients.

1.4 Teratogenicity: The Medication Review

Many cardiac drugs harm the developing fetus. You must switch these medications before conception.

ACE Inhibitors / ARBs (e.g., Ramipril, Losartan): These are toxic to fetal kidneys. They must be stopped.

Warfarin: This is the great dilemma. Warfarin causes embryopathy (bone defects) in the first trimester. However, it is the best drug for preventing clots in mechanical valves.

The 2026 Approach: We engage in "Shared Decision Making." If the warfarin dose is low (<5mg), some mothers choose to stay on it to protect their valve, accepting a small fetal risk. Others switch to Heparin (injections) which does not cross the placenta but is harder to manage and carries higher risk of valve failure for the mother.

1.5 The Delivery Plan

The liaison with the obstetrician is vital here. A common misconception is that all heart patients need a Caesarean section (C-section). This is false.

Vaginal Delivery is Preferred: It results in less blood loss and fewer infection risks than a C-section. We use an epidural to minimize pain and tachycardia. We often use an "assisted second stage" (forceps or vacuum) so the mother does not have to strain (Valsalva), which strains the heart.

When is C-Section Mandatory?

Preterm labor while on full anticoagulation (to prevent fetal brain bleed).

Severe aortic pathology (risk of dissection).

Severe Pulmonary Hypertension (mWHO IV).

Part 2: Multi-Specialty Liaison (Subtopic 7.4)

2.1 The Cardiologist as Gatekeeper

ACHD patients get appendicitis, break hips, and develop cancer just like anyone else. When they need non-cardiac surgery, the non-cardiac teams (surgeons, anesthetists) will panic. They will look to you for leadership.

Your role is to translate "cardiac anatomy" into "anesthetic risk."

2.2 Assessing Risk for Non-Cardiac Surgery

The risk is rarely the surgery itself; it is the anesthesia and the fluid shifts.

The Threat of Hypotension: Induction of anesthesia causes vasodilation (widening of blood vessels). In a patient with a fixed obstruction (like severe aortic stenosis), this drop in pressure means the heart cannot push blood to the brain. Cardiac arrest can occur on induction.

The Threat of the Shunt: In patients with a "hole in the heart" (ASD/VSD), bubbles of air in an IV line are deadly. In a normal person, a tiny air bubble goes to the lungs and is filtered out. In an ACHD patient, the bubble can cross the hole, travel to the brain, and cause a stroke.

Actionable Advice: You must instruct the anesthetist to use air filters on all IV lines for ACHD patients.

2.3 Anticoagulation Management: The Bridging Dilemma

Managing blood thinners during surgery is a high-stakes balancing act.

Mechanical Valves: You cannot stop Warfarin for long. The valve will clot.

The Protocol: Stop Warfarin 3-5 days pre-op. When the INR drops, start a "bridge" of Low Molecular Weight Heparin (LMWH) or Unfractionated Heparin infusion. Stop the Heparin 4-6 hours before surgery. Restart it as soon as bleeding risk is controlled.

Fontan Patients: These patients rely on passive blood flow to the lungs. They clot easily, but they also bleed easily due to liver congestion. Bridging them requires an expert hematologist and ACHD cardiologist working together.

2.4 Endocarditis Prophylaxis: The Guidelines

Infective Endocarditis (IE) is a devastating infection of the heart lining.

The UK (NICE) vs. The World (ESC/AHA): This is a specific point of friction in the UK curriculum.

NICE Guidelines (UK): Historically, they advised against routine antibiotic prophylaxis for dental procedures, citing lack of evidence.

ESC Guidelines (Europe): They strongly recommend prophylaxis for high-risk patients (prosthetic valves, previous endocarditis, cyanotic heart disease).

The 2026 Reality: Most UK cardiologists now follow the ESC approach for high-risk patients, viewing the risk of death from endocarditis as far worse than the risk of antibiotic reaction. You must document this decision clearly. "Given high-risk anatomy, antibiotic prophylaxis is recommended in line with ESC standards."

2.5 Anaesthetic Risks in Specific Lesions

You must tailor your advice to the lesion:

Eisenmenger Syndrome (PAH): This is the highest risk group. A drop in blood pressure can be fatal. Spinal anesthesia (which drops BP massively) is often contraindicated. General anesthesia must be managed by a senior cardiac anesthetist.

Fontan Circulation: These patients depend on "preload" (fluid status). If they are dehydrated (NBM for surgery) and then anesthetized, their cardiac output crashes. They need careful pre-loading with IV fluids before anesthesia starts.

Tetralogy of Fallot: Watch for the Right Ventricle. If they have severe pulmonary regurgitation, the RV is dilated and weak. Fluid overload can tip them into right heart failure.

Core Theme: Heart Failure

8.1 Diagnosis and Aetiology Assessment

The diagnosis of heart failure is a clinical puzzle. It relies on a triad: typical symptoms, specific signs, and objective evidence of structural or functional cardiac abnormality.

The Clinical Presentation: Symptoms and Signs

The classic presentation remains the breathless patient. However, the nuance lies in distinguishing cardiac breathlessness from respiratory causes.

Breathlessness (Dyspnoea): This is often exertional initially. As the ventricle stiffens or dilates, pressures rise in the left atrium, transmitting back to the pulmonary capillaries, causing interstitial oedema. This explains orthopnoea (breathlessness when lying flat) and Paroxysmal Nocturnal Dyspnoea (PND)—waking up gasping for air.

Fatigue: Often overlooked, this is a sign of "forward failure"—inadequate perfusion of skeletal muscles.

Oedema: Peripheral oedema is the hallmark of right-sided congestion. However, in 2026 practice, we recognize that visible oedema is a late sign. Trainees must look for "subclinical congestion" (elevated jugular venous pressure, hepatomegaly) before the ankles swell.

Clinical Pearl: In elderly patients, "confusion" or "reduced exercise tolerance" may be the only sign of heart failure, as they may not be active enough to experience classic exertional dyspnoea.

Investigating the Aetiology: The "Why"

Diagnosing "Heart Failure" is not a complete diagnosis; it is like diagnosing "fever." You must find the cause. The UK curriculum demands a rigorous hunt for the aetiology because it dictates the treatment.

Ischaemic Heart Disease (IHD): The most common cause. Previous myocardial infarctions scar the ventricle, leading to regional wall motion abnormalities (RWMA) and reduced contractility.

Valvular Heart Disease: Aortic stenosis (pressure overload) or mitral regurgitation (volume overload) can lead to ventricular remodeling.

Hypertension: Chronic high blood pressure forces the heart to pump against high resistance (afterload), causing Left Ventricular Hypertrophy (LVH). Eventually, the muscle stiffens (HFpEF) or burns out and dilates (HFrEF).

Dilated Cardiomyopathy (DCM): A diagnosis of exclusion, often familial or genetic.

Infiltrative Causes (The 2026 Focus): Amyloidosis (specifically ATTR-CM) is now diagnosed much more frequently thanks to better awareness. It presents with "red flags" like carpal tunnel syndrome, spinal stenosis, and a "sparkling" septum on echo.

Investigations: Characterizing the Myocardium

1. Natriuretic Peptides (NT-proBNP): This is the "rule-out" test. When the heart muscle stretches, it releases BNP. A normal level virtually excludes untreated heart failure. However, levels can be falsely low in obesity or falsely high in renal failure and atrial fibrillation.

2. Transthoracic Echocardiography (TTE): The workhorse of cardiology. It answers three key questions:

Structure: Are the valves working? Is the muscle thick (hypertrophy) or thin (dilation)?

Function: What is the Ejection Fraction (EF)? This classifies the patient into HFrEF (<40%), HFmrEF (41-49%), or HFpEF (≥ 50%).

Pressures: It estimates pulmonary artery pressures to screen for pulmonary hypertension.

3. Cardiac MRI (CMR): CMR is the gold standard for tissue characterization. While Echo sees the motion, MRI sees the tissue.

Scarring: Late Gadolinium Enhancement (LGE) can distinguish between ischaemic scarring (subendocardial) and non-ischaemic scarring (mid-wall or epicardial), which is crucial for determining aetiology in dilated cardiomyopathy.

Infiltration: It is definitive for diagnosing conditions like Sarcoidosis or Amyloidosis which may require specific enzyme replacement or immunosuppressive therapies.

Management of New-Onset Acute Heart Failure

When a patient presents acutely "wet" (congested), the immediate priority is decongestion.

Intravenous Diuretics: Furosemide is given intravenously to offload fluid. The 2026 standard involves early assessment of diuretic response (checking sodium in the urine) to escalate doses rapidly if the patient isn't responding ("diuretic resistance").

Vasodilators: Nitrates are used if the blood pressure is high to reduce the workload on the heart.

Oxygen/CPAP: Non-invasive ventilation is used if the patient is hypoxic and struggling to breathe, as it physically pushes fluid out of the alveoli.

8.2 Medical Optimization and Device Therapy

Once the patient is stable and "dry" (euvolemic), the focus shifts to prognostic medication. In 2026, the management of Heart Failure with Reduced Ejection Fraction (HFrEF) is one of the most evidence-based areas in all of medicine.

The Four Pillars of HFrEF Treatment

We no longer "step up" therapy slowly over months. The modern approach is the rapid sequencing or simultaneous initiation of the "Four Pillars." These drugs do not just treat symptoms; they fundamentally alter the biology of the failing heart and prolong life.

1. Beta-Blockers (Bisoprolol, Carvedilol, Nebivolol):

Mechanism: They block the sympathetic nervous system (adrenaline). In heart failure, the body is in a constant "fight or flight" mode, whipping the tired heart to beat faster. Beta-blockers slow the heart, protecting it from toxic catecholamines and reducing arrhythmia risk.

Clinical Tip: Start low and go slow. They can initially make patients feel tired.

2. RAAS Inhibitors (ACEi / ARNI):

ACE Inhibitors (Ramipril, Enalapril): Block the production of Angiotensin II, a potent vasoconstrictor that clamps down on arteries and causes salt retention.

ARNI (Sacubitril/Valsartan): Now the preferred first-line over ACEi in many 2026 guidelines for symptomatic patients. It combines a RAAS blocker with a Neprilysin inhibitor. Neprilysin breaks down good natriuretic peptides; inhibiting it boosts the body's natural "offloading" system.

3. Mineralocorticoid Receptor Antagonists (MRA - Spironolactone, Eplerenone):

Mechanism: They block Aldosterone. Aldosterone causes fibrosis (scarring) of the heart muscle and salt retention. Blocking it prevents the heart from becoming stiff and reduces sudden cardiac death.

Monitoring: Vital to watch Potassium (K^+) and renal function.

4. SGLT2 Inhibitors (Dapagliflozin, Empagliflozin):

Mechanism: Originally diabetes drugs, these are now pure heart failure drugs. They encourage glucose and sodium excretion in urine (osmotic diuresis) and improve myocardial energetics (how the heart uses fuel).

The 2026 Status: They are mandatory for HFrEF and are now the only class firmly established to help HFpEF (Preserved Ejection Fraction) as well.

New and Emerging Therapies (2026 Updates)

Beyond the pillars, specific scenarios require "add-on" therapies:

Vericiguat: A soluble guanylate cyclase stimulator used in high-risk patients who have recently been hospitalized despite good therapy.

Omecamtiv Mecarbil: A cardiac myosin activator that increases the duration of contraction without increasing oxygen demand. It is reserved for severe HFrEF where blood pressure is too low for other drugs.

GLP-1 Agonists (Semaglutide): In 2026, these are strongly recommended for the obese HFpEF phenotype to reduce symptoms and inflammation.

Device Therapy: ICD and CRT

Medical therapy has limits. When the Ejection Fraction remains low (<35%) despite optimal drugs for 3 months, we consider devices.

1. Implantable Cardioverter Defibrillator (ICD):

The Risk: Patients with HFrEF are at high risk of sudden death from Ventricular Tachycardia (VT) or Fibrillation (VF).

The Solution: An ICD monitors the rhythm and delivers a shock to reset the heart if it detects a lethal arrhythmia. It acts as an airbag—it doesn't prevent the crash, but it saves the life.

2. Cardiac Resynchronization Therapy (CRT):

The Problem: In many HF patients, the electrical wiring is damaged (Left Bundle Branch Block - LBBB). This causes the left and right ventricles to beat out of sync (dyssynchrony), causing the heart to wobble rather than squeeze.

The Solution: CRT uses an extra lead placed via the coronary sinus to pace the left ventricle directly. This resynchronizes the contraction, often improving the EF and symptoms dramatically.

Nuance in Co-morbidities: The Renal Challenge

One of the hardest skills for a trainee is managing heart failure in the context of Chronic Kidney Disease (CKD). This is often called "Cardiorenal Syndrome."

The Bump in Creatinine: When starting ACEi/ARNI or SGLT2i, the filtration pressure in the kidney drops, causing a rise in creatinine. In 2026, we accept a rise of up to 30-50% without stopping the drug. This is often a "hemodynamic" change, not true kidney damage.

Hyperkalaemia: MRAs raise potassium. Modern potassium binders (Patiromer, Sodium Zirconium Cyclosilicate) allow us to keep patients on life-saving MRAs even if their potassium runs high, a major shift from historical practice where we would simply stop the drug.

2. Module 8.3: Pulmonary Hypertension and Pericardial Disease

The management of the pulmonary vasculature and the pericardium represents a collision of hemodynamics and inflammation. As per the UK curriculum, the trainee must move beyond basic identification to expert management and procedural independence.

2.1. Pulmonary Hypertension (PH): The Silent Right Heart Killer

Pulmonary hypertension is often described as the "Cinderella" of cardiology—frequently ignored until the stroke of midnight when right heart failure sets in. By 2026, our understanding has shifted from treating pressures to treating the phenotype.

The Assessment and Diagnosis Paradigm The curriculum mandates a strict ability to differentiate between the five clinical groups of PH. This is not academic pedantry; it is a matter of life and death, as therapies for Group 1 (PAH) can kill a patient with Group 2 (Left Heart Disease) PH.

Echocardiography as the Gatekeeper: The trainee must look beyond the estimated Pulmonary Artery Systolic Pressure (PASP). We now focus on the "TR velocity" signal reliability and, crucially, the coupling of the right ventricle (RV) to the pulmonary circulation (TAPSE/PASP ratios).

The Gold Standard: Right Heart Catheterization (RHC): You cannot diagnose PH without invasive hemodynamics. The definition has tightened in recent years (mPAP > 20 mmHg). The trainee must be adept at interpreting the pulmonary vascular resistance (PVR) and the pulmonary capillary wedge pressure (PCWP). A wedge pressure >15 mmHg immediately shunts the patient into the "post-capillary" world of left heart failure, drastically changing the management plan.

The National Centre Imperative A critical competency is knowing when to let go. Pulmonary Arterial Hypertension (PAH) and Chronic Thromboembolic Pulmonary

Hypertension (CTEPH) are rare diseases. The curriculum requires trainees to refer these patients to designated National Specialist Centres (e.g., in the UK context, centres like Hammersmith, Papworth, or Sheffield).

Why? Because the therapeutic arsenal has exploded. We are no longer just using PDE5 inhibitors (Sildenafil). We are utilizing triple combination therapies, subcutaneous prostacyclins, and novel activin signaling inhibitors that reverse remodeling. Furthermore, CTEPH is the only potentially curable form of heart failure via Pulmonary Endarterectomy (PEA). Missing this referral is a failure of care.

2.2. Pericardial Disease: Inflammation and Constraint

The 2025 ESC Guidelines on "Inflammatory Myocardial and Pericardial Syndromes" (IMPS) have revolutionized this subtopic. The pericardium is no longer viewed as a passive sac but as an active, inflammatory organ.

Pericarditis: The Fire Acute pericarditis is the most common form. The classic "saddle-shaped" ST elevation is helpful, but the diagnosis is clinical. The "2026 approach" emphasizes the use of Cardiac MRI (CMR) early in doubtful cases to assess for concomitant myocarditis (perimyocarditis), which changes exercise restrictions for athletes. Treatment remains anchored in high-dose NSAIDs and Colchicine, but the use of IL-1 blockers (like anakinra) for recurrent, refractory cases is now entering mainstream specialist thinking.

Constriction: The Vice Constrictive Pericarditis is the heart's "stiff jacket." It mimics liver failure and restrictive cardiomyopathy. The trainee must demonstrate the ability to identify "ventricular interdependence"—the phenomenon where the septum bounces into the left ventricle during inspiration because the heart is trapped in a fixed volume. Recognizing this on an echo (respiratory variation in mitral inflow >25%) triggers the referral for pericardiectomy, a high-risk but high-reward surgery.

2.3. Procedural Competency: Pericardiocentesis (Level 4)

The curriculum explicitly demands that a trainee be an independent operator (Level 4) for pericardiocentesis. This is a high-stakes procedure.

The Scenario: A patient presents with hypotension, muffled heart sounds, and distended neck veins (Beck's Triad). The echo shows a swinging heart and RA/RV collapse in diastole. This is tamponade. The pressure in the pericardium has exceeded the filling pressure of the heart.

The Technique: Blind subxiphoid approaches are relics of the past (unless during cardiac arrest). The standard of care is Echo-Guided Pericardiocentesis.

Step 1: Locate the largest fluid pocket closest to the skin (often apical or parasternal).

Step 2: Confirm the trajectory is free of lung or liver.

Step 3: Advance the needle under negative pressure.

Step 4: Use agitated saline (bubble study) to confirm the needle is in the sac, not the ventricle.

Safety: The trainee must know when not to tap. A dissection with tamponade requires a surgeon, not a needle.

3. Module 8.4: Palliative Care and Advanced Therapies

As we move to Module 8.4, the tone shifts from "fixing" to "managing." Heart failure has a malignant trajectory, often worse than many cancers. The curriculum requires a schizophrenic skill set: the ability to aggressively pursue life-extending technology (Transplant/LVAD) while simultaneously preparing for the end of life.

3.1. Advanced Heart Failure Therapies: The "Bridge" Concept

Identifying the "tipping point" is the hardest skill in cardiology. Trainees must recognize when conventional "Four Pillar" medical therapy (Beta-blockers, ARNI, MRA, SGLT2i) has failed. We use the INTERMACS profiles to classify these patients, ranging from "Crash and Burn" (Profile 1) to "Walking Wounded" (Profile 4-7).

Left Ventricular Assist Devices (LVADs) By 2026, LVADs are sophisticated, fully magnetically levitated centrifugal pumps (like the HeartMate 3 lineage). They are no longer just a "bridge to transplant" but increasingly a "destination therapy" for those ineligible for new hearts.

Trainee Responsibility: You must identify patients before right ventricular failure sets in. Once the RV fails, an LVAD is often futile because it relies on the RV to fill it.

Referral Criteria: Inability to walk one block (NYHA IV), intolerance to ACE inhibitors due to hypotension, and escalating diuretic doses.

Cardiac Transplantation This remains the gold standard, but it is a resource-constrained lottery. The trainee's role is referral timing. Refer too early, and the risk of the surgery outweighs the benefit. Refer too late, and irreversible pulmonary hypertension or renal failure (Cardiorenal syndrome) precludes the patient from the list.

3.2. Palliative Care: The "One Chance to Get it Right"

In the UK curriculum, palliative care is not "giving up"; it is "supportive care." The trajectory of heart failure is unpredictable—a "sawtooth" decline of decompensations followed by partial recoveries, until a sudden death or final dip occurs.

Symptom Control

Breathlessness: This is the most terrifying symptom. The trainee must be comfortable prescribing low-dose opioids (e.g., Morphine or Oxycodone) which reduce the sensation of air hunger without significantly depressing respiratory drive in tolerant patients.

The ICD Dilemma: A specific curricular requirement is the discussion of ICD Deactivation. There is nothing more undignified than a dying patient receiving high-voltage shocks for a terminal rhythm. Trainees must initiate "Advance Care Planning" (ACP) discussions early, ensuring that the device's shock function is turned off while pacing continues, allowing for a peaceful natural death.

Collaborative Care We must integrate with community heart failure nurses and palliative specialists. The "hospice" model is often underutilized in HF because patients are unpredictable. Therefore, much of this care happens at home. The 2026 cardiologist acts as the conductor, ensuring that diuretics are possibly converted to subcutaneous infusions if oral absorption fails (gut edema), and that the focus shifts from "prolonging life" to "optimizing quality."

Advanced Theme: Leading a Coronary Intervention Service

9.1 Complex Angiography and Physiology

This subtopic requires you to move beyond simple diagnostic pictures. You are now expected to perform comprehensive assessments that drive the "Heart Team" decision-making process.

Vascular Access: The "Radial First" Reality

By ST6, radial access should be your default. It is safer, cleaner, and preferred by patients. However, the curriculum demands you remain competent in femoral access. Why? Because complex large-bore procedures (like TAVI or Impella-supported PCI) often demand it.

The 2026 Standard: You must demonstrate independent proficiency in left heart catheterization via both radial and femoral routes.

The Trap: Do not lose your femoral skills. If a radial artery goes into spasm or the anatomy is tortuous, you must switch to femoral access without hesitation.

Technical Tip: Use ultrasound guidance for femoral punctures. It is no longer optional; it is the standard of care to reduce bleeding complications.

Invasive Physiology: FFR and iFR

We no longer stent based on "eyeball" estimation. Visual assessment of intermediate lesions is notoriously inaccurate. You must use invasive physiology to prove ischaemia before you treat.

Fractional Flow Reserve (FFR): This remains the gold standard for many. It requires adenosine to induce hyperaemia (maximum blood flow). A value of $\leqslant$0.80 indicates significant ischaemia.

Instantaneous Wave-Free Ratio (iFR): This is the adenosine-free alternative. It measures the pressure drop during the "wave-free period" of diastole. A value of $\leqslant$0.89 is the treatment cutoff.

The "New" Evidence (2026 Perspective): Recent 5-year follow-up data from major trials (like DEFINE-FLAIR) has solidified the standing of iFR. We now know that iFR-guided outcomes are statistically comparable to FFR-guided outcomes in the long term.

Clinical Application: If a patient has severe asthma or simply cannot tolerate the chest tightness caused by adenosine, use iFR. It is faster and equally safe.

Discordance: Occasionally, FFR and iFR disagree. In these cases, trust the physiology that best matches the patient's clinical presentation.

Intracoronary Imaging: IVUS and OCT

This is the era of "Precision PCI." Angiography gives you a 2D silhouette of a 3D tube. It lies to you. Intracoronary imaging tells the truth. The 2024/2025 ESC Guidelines have elevated the recommendation for imaging in complex lesions to Class I.

1. Intravascular Ultrasound (IVUS):

Strengths: It sees deep. It can see through blood (no contrast needed for the flush). It is ideal for ostial lesions (where the guide catheter hides the view) and Left Main Stem (LMS) disease.

Key Metric: For LMS disease, we look for a Minimum Lumen Area (MLA) of >6.0 mm2. Anything less is often functionally significant.

2. Optical Coherence Tomography (OCT):

Strengths: It has 10x the resolution of IVUS. It uses light, not sound. It produces beautiful, near-histological images.

Best For: Seeing thrombus, checking stent apposition (is the stent touching the wall?), and characterizing plaque morphology (calcium vs. lipid).

Limitation: It requires a blood-free field, meaning you must inject contrast. Avoid it in patients with severe renal failure.

The Heart Team Meeting

You are the eyes of the surgeons. When you perform a diagnostic angiogram on a complex patient, you are gathering intelligence for the Heart Team.

The Syntax Score: You must be able to calculate this. It quantifies the anatomical complexity of the disease.

Low Score (0-22): PCI is usually equal to surgery.

High Score (>33): Coronary Artery Bypass Graft (CABG) is usually superior, especially in diabetics.

Frailty: Anatomy is not destiny. A patient with a high Syntax score might still be turned down for surgery if they are "frail" or have a "porcelain aorta" (heavily calcified).

You must advocate for the best clinical option, not just the anatomical one.

9.2 Percutaneous Coronary Intervention (PCI)

This section is the core of your technical training. You must transition from "assisting" to "leading" procedures.
Stable vs. Acute Coronary Syndromes

Stable Angina: The goal is symptom relief. If the patient has no symptoms, we rarely stent just for the sake of it (unless it is Left Main or proximal LAD disease).

ACS (STEMI/NSTEMI): The goal is survival and myocardial salvage. Speed matters. You must be proficient in aspiration thrombectomy (sucking out the clot) and handling "no-reflow" (when the microvasculature gets plugged).

Complex Lesion Management

Simple lesions are rare in ST6. You will face the "big three" challenges:

1. Bifurcation Lesions: This is where a vessel splits. If you stent the main branch, you risk "jailing" (blocking) the side branch.

The Provisional Strategy: This is your default. Stent the main vessel, and only touch the side branch if it gets into trouble. "Keep it simple" is the mantra.

Two-Stent Strategies (DK Crush / Culotte): You need these for true bifurcations where both branches are large and diseased. The "DK Crush" technique has superior data (from the DKCRUSH trials) for Left Main bifurcations.

2. Calcific Disease: Calcium is the enemy of the stent. If you deploy a stent into a rock-hard ring of calcium, it will not expand ("underexpansion"). This is a leading cause of stent failure (restenosis or thrombosis).

Rotational Atherectomy (Rotablation): A diamond-tipped burr drills through the calcium. It is aggressive but effective for "un-crossable" lesions.

Intravascular Lithotripsy (IVL): This technology uses sonic pressure waves to crack deep calcium without damaging the soft tissue. It is the "gentler" option and has become a workhorse in UK labs by 2026. Think of it as breaking up a kidney stone, but inside the artery.

3. Coronary Bypass Grafts: Vein grafts are fragile. They are often filled with friable, cheesy plaque. Stenting them carries a high risk of distal embolization (debris floating downstream and causing a heart attack).

Strategy: Use embolic protection devices (filters) when possible. Or better yet, try to open the native artery instead of fixing the old graft.

Chronic Total Occlusions (CTO)

A CTO is an artery that has been 100% blocked for more than 3 months.

The Decision: Just because it is closed does not mean you must open it. We treat CTOs for symptoms (angina), not just for cosmetics.

The Skillset: You need to understand "dual injection" (shooting contrast into both left and right arteries simultaneously to see the collateral flow). You must learn when to refer these cases to a dedicated CTO operator.

Section 1: Primary PCI and Haemodynamic Support (Subtopic 9.3)

This section requires you to move beyond the technical "diagnosis-to-wire" reflex and engage with complex physiology. You are now the decision-maker at 3:00 AM.

1. The Modern Primary PCI (PPCI) Rota

Participation in the PPCI rota is the crucible of interventional training. By 2026, the focus has shifted from simple door-to-balloon times to "total system performance."

The Clinical Reality: You aren't just treating an artery; you are treating a syndrome. In a standard STEMI (ST-Elevation Myocardial Infarction), your role is efficiency. But in the "shocked" patient, your role is strategy.

The "Shock Team" Concept: Following the 2025 updates to ESC and BCIS guidelines, we now emphasize the "Shock Team." You must demonstrate the ability to activate and coordinate this multi-disciplinary group—involving intensivists, heart failure specialists, and sometimes cardiac surgeons—before you even puncture the femoral artery.

2. Management of Haemodynamic Instability

When a patient crashes on the table, the old algorithms often fail. You need a nuanced understanding of pressure versus flow.

Pharmacological Support (The Chemical Bridge) You must show competence in mixing and titrating vasoactive drugs independently.

Vasopressors: Norepinephrine (Noradrenaline) remains our workhorse. It tightens the vessels to maintain perfusion pressure to the brain and heart. In 2026, we are quicker to add Vasopressin in refractory shock to avoid the toxic effects of high-dose catecholamines.

Inotropes: When the heart muscle is stunned, Dobutamine or Milrinone is used. However, you must balance the "squeeze" against the "burn"—these drugs increase oxygen demand in an already starving heart. The advanced trainee knows when to stop whipping the tired horse and move to mechanical support.

Mechanical Circulatory Support (MCS): The 2026 Paradigm Shift This is where the biggest changes have occurred in recent years.

The Decline of the IABP: The Intra-Aortic Balloon Pump (IABP), once a staple, is now largely a Class III (harm/no benefit) intervention for routine cardiogenic shock. You should only use it for specific mechanical complications (like a hole in the heart muscle—VSD) or if no other option exists. If you reach for an IABP in 2026 for a standard shock case without justification, you will fail the audit.

The Rise of Impella (Micro-axial Flow Pumps): Following the DanGer Shock trial data solidified in late 2024/2025, the Impella device has seen a conditional upgrade. It actively unloads the left ventricle (unlike ECMO, which increases afterload). Your training must verify your ability to position this device across the aortic valve safely. It sucks blood from the ventricle and ejects it into the aorta, doing the heart's work for it.

VA-ECMO: Veno-Arterial Extracorporeal Membrane Oxygenation is the "nuclear option." It replaces both heart and lung function. However, the ECLS-SHOCK trial taught us that early, routine use doesn't save lives in all comers. It is now reserved for "salvage" or young patients as a bridge to transplant.

3. Cardiac Arrest Survivors: To Angio or Not?

A major learning point for 9.3 is the management of the post-cardiac arrest patient who has a pulse (ROSC) but is in a coma.

The Rule: If the ECG shows STEMI, you go to the lab immediately.

The Nuance: If the ECG does not show STEMI, the 2026 guidelines (based on the TOMAHAWK and COACT trials) say stop. Do not rush to the cath lab. These patients need intensive care (cooling, neurological protection) first. Rushing them to angiography often destabilizes them without fixing the root cause. You must be confident enough to turn the ambulance away from the lab and towards the ICU.

Section 2: Service Leadership and Safety (Subtopic 9.4)

An advanced trainee is an "Acting Consultant." This means you are responsible for the ecosystem of the lab, not just the patient on the table.

1. Radiation Safety: Protecting the Future

Ionising radiation is the silent killer in our profession. In 2026, the "ALARA" principle (As Low As Reasonably Achievable) is strictly enforced by the CQC (Care Quality Commission).

The New Tech: We now utilize AI-driven noise reduction software that allows us to work at ultra-low frame rates (3-4 frames per second) without losing image quality.

Zero-Gravity Suits: You may see "suspended" lead suits in modern labs to save your spine.

The Leadership Role: You are responsible for the junior staff. If a nurse or radiographer steps inside the "isocenter" (the high-dose zone) without protection, it is your job to stop the procedure. You must also monitor "Air Kerma" (skin dose) to prevent radiation burns on patients during long procedures (like CTOs).

2. Quality Control and Audit

In the UK NHS, "if it isn't recorded, it didn't happen."

BCIS Audit: Every single stent deployed in the UK is entered into the BCIS (British Cardiovascular Intervention Society) database. You must ensure your data is accurate.

M&M Meetings: You must lead Morbidity and Mortality meetings. This isn't about blaming; it's about system learning. If a patient died, was it the anatomy? Or was it a delay in transfer? Or a missing piece of kit?

Outcome Tracking: We no longer just track survival. We track "quality of life" and "angina-free status."

3. Resource Allocation and The "Bed Crisis"

This is the most "human" skill of all. The NHS operates under constant pressure.

The Scenario: You have one clean lab and one staffed recovery bed. You have three patients:

A stable angina patient who has waited 18 months.

An NSTEMI patient with chest pain.

A "Code Primary" (STEMI) 10 minutes away.

The Decision: The advanced trainee must make the call. You cancel the elective (empathizing with their frustration), you hold the NSTEMI, and you keep the room open for the STEMI. Managing the friction this causes—with management, bed managers, and angry relatives—is the true test of your leadership.

Advanced Theme: Leading a Cardiac Imaging Service

10.1 Multi-Modality Expertise and Strategy

The Philosophy of Strategic Imaging

Imaging is not just about taking pictures. It is about answering a clinical question with the lowest risk and highest accuracy. This subtopic requires you to move beyond "working knowledge." You must become an authority.

When a patient presents with heart failure, what is your first move? Do you order an Echo? A CMR? A nuclear scan? The answer depends on the patient, not just the technology.

In 2026, we focus on the "appropriate use criteria." You must learn to weigh the benefits of different techniques. For example, MRI is the gold standard for tissue characterization. It sees fibrosis that Echo misses. However, Nuclear Medicine (SPECT/PET) remains superior for specific viability questions in patients with metal devices who cannot have an MRI.

Comparative Modalities: The Matrix of Choice

To be an expert, you must understand the strengths of each tool.

Echocardiography (Echo): This is the bedside workhorse. It is fast, safe, and portable. It gives unbeatable temporal resolution (frame rate). It is the primary tool for haemodynamics (blood flow) and valve assessment. However, it struggles with "poor acoustic windows" (e.g., in patients with lung disease or obesity).

Cardiovascular Magnetic Resonance (CMR): This is the king of anatomy and tissue. In 2026, CMR is the definitive test for cardiomyopathies. It can differentiate between ischaemic (heart attack) scarring and non-ischaemic fibrosis (like myocarditis). It uses no radiation. Its main drawback is availability and patient claustrophobia.

Cardiac Computed Tomography (CCT): CCT has revolutionized chest pain clinics. It is the best tool for excluding coronary artery disease. With the new 2026 photon-counting scanners, we can now see inside stents and heavily calcified arteries with incredible clarity. It uses radiation, though doses are now very low.

Nuclear Cardiology (SPECT/PET): While less common for anatomy, this is vital for physiology. It shows us metabolism. PET scans are critical for diagnosing infective endocarditis on valves when other scans are inconclusive. It is also the arbiter for cardiac sarcoidosis.

Clinical Scenario: Viability Assessment

Let us look at a real-world example. A patient has a blocked artery and a weak heart muscle. The surgeon asks: "Is the muscle dead, or is it just hibernating?" If it is dead, bypass surgery is useless. If it is hibernating, surgery will restore function.

The CMR Approach: You look for "Late Gadolinium Enhancement" (LGE). If the scar is thin (less than 50% of the wall), the tissue is viable. This is an anatomical answer.

The Stress Echo Approach: You give Dobutamine. You watch the wall. If it thickens during low-dose stress, it is alive. This is a functional answer.

The Nuclear Approach: You look for metabolic activity. Even if the muscle is not moving, if it "eats" the tracer, it is alive.

As a multi-modality expert, you must choose the right test. If the patient has a pacemaker that is not MRI-conditional, you choose Echo or Nuclear. If the image quality on Echo is poor, you move to Nuclear. This decision-making process is the core of Subtopic 10.1.

10.2 Advanced Echocardiography Services

The Requirement for Mastery

For those of you choosing Echocardiography as your primary specialty, the bar is set high. You are not just a scanner. You are the safeguard of the department.

You must be able to perform and supervise Transoesophageal Echocardiography (TOE), Stress Echocardiography, and 3D techniques. You must also be ready to lead. This means managing workflows, auditing report quality, and teaching junior fellows.

Transoesophageal Echocardiography (TOE)

TOE involves passing a probe down the oesophagus. It sits directly behind the heart. The views are crystal clear.

Safety and Sedation: You must be competent in conscious sedation. You need to manage the patient's airway and comfort. You must know the contraindications, such as oesophageal strictures or varices. In 2026, safety checklists are mandatory before every procedure.

Structural Planning: TOE is the map for the surgeon. If a patient needs a mitral valve repair, you must tell the surgeon exactly which scallop of the valve is prolapsing. Is it P2? Is it A2? Your report guides their scalpel.

Interventional Guidance: During procedures like a TAVI (aortic valve replacement) or MitraClip, you are the "eyes" of the team. You guide the catheter in real-time.

Stress Echocardiography

Stress echo is a dynamic test. You make the heart work hard and watch for failure.

Exercise vs. Pharmacological: The preferred method is exercise (treadmill or bike) because it is physiological. It mimics real life. However, for patients who cannot walk, we use Dobutamine to simulate exercise.

The Ischaemic Cascade: You are looking for "wall motion abnormalities." When a coronary artery is blocked, the wall it feeds stops thickening before the patient feels pain and before the ECG changes. This makes stress echo incredibly sensitive.

Valvular Stress: We also use this for valves. A valve might look "moderate" at rest but become "severe" when the patient runs. This is critical for timing surgery in asymptomatic patients.

3D Echocardiography

Two decades ago, 3D echo was a gimmick. In 2026, it is a requirement.

Volume Assessment: 2D echo relies on geometric assumptions (mathematical guesses) to calculate heart volume. 3D echo measures the actual volume, voxel by voxel. It is as accurate as MRI.

The "Surgeon's View": With 3D, you can rotate the valve on the screen to show the surgeon exactly what they will see in the operating theatre. This "en face" view is mandatory for planning complex repairs.

The Heart Team and Departmental Leadership

The curriculum places heavy emphasis on your role in the "Heart Team."

This is a multidisciplinary meeting. It includes surgeons, interventionists, and imagers. You are the voice of the anatomy. When they debate whether to fix a valve with a clip or a surgery, they turn to you. You must explain the complex pathology simply and clearly.

You are also responsible for Quality Assurance (QA). You must regularly audit the reports of your department. Are the measurements accurate? Is the conclusion supported by the data? You must provide feedback to sonographers and registrars to maintain high standards.

2026 Update: The Future is Now

Since the writing of the original curriculum, technology has surged forward. To be a top-tier trainee in 2026, you must be aware of these advancements.

Artificial Intelligence (AI) Integration

In 2026, AI is not about replacing the doctor. It is about removing the drudgery.

Automated Strain: We now use AI to automatically calculate "Global Longitudinal Strain" (GLS). This detects subtle heart failure years before the ejection fraction drops. The AI draws the contours instantly, reducing variability between different observers.

Workflow Triage: Smart algorithms now pre-read scans. They flag "normal" scans for a quick review and prioritize "abnormal" scans for urgent attention. This helps manage the massive waiting lists in the NHS.

Fusion Imaging

We are increasingly merging modalities. We can now overlay a CT scan onto a live fluoroscopy screen in the cath lab. This allows the interventionist to see the calcium and the soft tissue simultaneously while placing a valve. As an imaging specialist, you are the one who registers and aligns these datasets.

Photon-Counting CT

This is the cutting edge. Traditional CT detectors measure the energy of X-rays. Photon-counting detectors count the individual particles of light.

This gives us images with vastly higher resolution and less noise. It allows us to subtract calcium from the image digitally, letting us see the artery lumen underneath heavy calcification. This was impossible just five years ago.

2. Subtopic 10.3: Cross-Sectional Imaging (CT and CMR)

This section defines the rigorous standards required to lead a Computed Tomography (CT) or Cardiovascular Magnetic Resonance (CMR) service. It is not enough to simply "read" scans. You must own the service.

2.1. The Independent Reporter: Mastery of Complexity

To function as a consultant reporter, you must move beyond the basics. A Level 2 or Level 3 accreditation (such as from the BSCI or EACVI) is the benchmark. This signifies that you can handle the "grey areas" where binary answers do not exist.

Myocardial Viability and Ischaemia In CMR, assessing viability is a cornerstone skill. You are looking for "late gadolinium enhancement" (LGE). This tells us if the muscle is dead (scarred) or hibernating.

Example: Consider a patient with chronic heart failure and severe triple-vessel disease. The surgeon needs to know: "If I bypass these vessels, will the muscle recover?" You must be able to quantify the transmurality of the scar. If the scar is less than 50% of the wall thickness, revascularization might save the patient. If it is full-thickness (transmural), surgery is futile risk. Your report guides that life-altering decision.

Infiltrative Diseases The detection of infiltrative diseases like Cardiac Amyloidosis has revolutionized heart failure management in the last few years.

Example: A patient presents with "heart failure with preserved ejection fraction" (HFpEF). Their echo shows thick walls. Is it hypertension? Or is it Amyloid? On CMR, you must look for the characteristic "global subendocardial enhancement" and abnormal T1 mapping values. In 2026, with new therapies available for Amyloidosis, missing this diagnosis is no longer acceptable. You must be able to spot the subtle "nulling" patterns that suggest the myocardium is infiltrated with abnormal protein.

Congenital Anatomy Adult Congenital Heart Disease (ACHD) is becoming more common as patients survive childhood repairs. You don't need to be a congenital super-specialist, but you must recognize the anatomy.

Example: A young patient presents with right heart dilation. You must be able to trace the pulmonary veins on a CT or MRI. Are they draining correctly into the left atrium? Or is there a Sinus Venosus defect draining into the SVC? You must identify these anomalous connections independently, without needing a second opinion for every case.

2.2. Service Leadership: Managing the Machine and the Team

Being a leader means taking responsibility for the entire ecosystem of the scanner. You are responsible for the safety of the patient and the quality of the image before the scan even begins.

Protocol Management You must decide how the scan is done. A "one-size-fits-all" approach fails in cardiac imaging.

Example: A patient with a high heart rate (e.g., 85 bpm) arrives for a CT Coronary Angiogram. A standard retrospective spiral scan would deliver a massive radiation dose. As the lead, you must establish protocols that dictate the use of beta-blockers to lower the rate. If that fails, you must know when to switch to a high-pitch "flash" mode (if your scanner supports it) or when to cancel the scan to avoid a non-diagnostic result. You are the gatekeeper of quality.

Contrast Safety You deal with two main types of contrast: Iodinated (for CT) and Gadolinium-based (for CMR). Both carry risks that you must manage.

Example: A diabetic patient with renal impairment needs a scan. For CT, you must calculate their eGFR. If it is borderline, do you proceed? You need a hydration protocol in place. For CMR, you must be aware of the rare but serious Nephrogenic Systemic Fibrosis (NSF), although modern agents have reduced this risk. You must ensure your department has a robust anaphylaxis drill. If a patient collapses on the table, the radiographers will look to you. You must lead the resuscitation.

Supervision of Radiographers Radiographers are your partners. They operate the scanner, but they rely on your clinical judgement.

Example: During a stress perfusion CMR, the patient develops a transient Mobitz II heart block. The radiographer might panic and want to stop. You need to be in the console room, calm and collected. You assess the rhythm. You decide if it is safe to complete the stress portion or if you need to administer Aminophylline to reverse the stressor. Your presence provides the safety net that allows the team to function.

3. Subtopic 10.4: Innovation and Education in Imaging

In 2026, technology moves faster than textbooks. This subtopic requires you to be forward-thinking. You must be an educator who bridges the gap between the pixel and the patient.

3.1. Identifying and Applying Novel Techniques

You must constantly scan the horizon for new tools that improve patient care. You cannot rely on the methods of 2020.

Photon-Counting CT By 2026, Photon-Counting CT has started to enter clinical practice. This is a game-changer. It counts individual X-ray photons, allowing for vastly better spatial resolution and "spectral" information.

Example: A patient has heavy calcification in their coronary arteries. On a standard CT, this calcium "blooms," hiding the lumen and making it impossible to rule out stenosis. With Photon-Counting CT, you can "subtract" the calcium or see through the blooming with higher resolution. As an advanced trainee, you should be advocating for this technology or understanding how to refer patients to centers that have it.

Artificial Intelligence (AI) in Workflow AI is not about replacing the doctor; it is about removing the drudgery.

Example: In a busy CMR list, drawing contours around the ventricle to calculate ejection fraction used to take 15 minutes per patient. Now, AI does it in 10 seconds. Your role is to validate the AI. Does the contour make sense? Did it mistake the papillary muscle for the wall? You must understand the limitations of the "black box" and ensure that automation does not lead to complacency.

3.2. The Imager as Educator

You are the ambassador for imaging within the cardiology department. Other colleagues (interventionalists, heart failure specialists) may not understand the nuances of what you do. You must teach them.

Leading Imaging Meetings (MDTs) The Multidisciplinary Team (MDT) meeting is where imaging proves its worth. You must present images clearly and concisely.

Example: In a valve MDT, the surgeons are discussing a TAVI (Transcatheter Aortic Valve Implantation). They need to know the annular size. You don't just read the number; you show them the 3D reconstruction of the aorta. You demonstrate the distance to the coronary ostia. You explain why a certain valve size might occlude the coronary artery. You are teaching the team why the anatomy matters.

Teaching Core Trainees You must mentor the next generation. Core trainees need to understand the "appropriate use criteria"—knowing when to order a test is as important as knowing how to report it.

Example: A junior doctor orders a cardiac CT for a patient with a high pre-test probability of ischaemia and a known allergy to iodine. This is a poor choice. You don't just reject the request. You sit them down. You explain that a stress echo or stress MRI would be safer and more diagnostic. You teach them the logic of modality selection, ensuring they become better clinicians.

4. Deep Dive Analysis: The Integration of Skills

The true expert integrates these subtopics. You do not just "do a CT" or "teach a class." You combine leadership, innovation, and clinical acumen.

Consider the "One-Stop Shop" Chest Pain Clinic, a model prevalent in 2026.

The Scenario: A patient walks in with atypical chest pain.

The Imaging Role: You have set up a protocol where they get a calcium score immediately. If it is zero and they are low risk, they go home. If it is high, they move to CT Angiography (CCTA) or Functional Imaging (FFR-CT).

The Innovation: You use AI-driven FFR-CT (Fractional Flow Reserve) to determine if a narrowing is actually restricting blood flow, saving the patient an invasive angiogram.

The Education: You review this case with the junior fellows later, showing them how the non-invasive test altered the management plan.

Advanced Theme: Leading an Arrhythmia Service

Chapter 1: The Diagnostic EP Study—The Foundation of Logic

Before we burn or freeze any tissue, we must understand the mechanism. The diagnostic EP study is the bedrock of our specialty. It is a deductive logic puzzle played out in real-time within the human heart.

1.1 The Setup: "Zero-Fluoro" by Default In the past, EP was done in grayscale under heavy X-ray. Today, in 2026, our default is "Zero-Fluoroscopy." You will learn to rely on 3D Electro-anatomical Mapping (EAM) systems—think of them as the GPS of the heart—rather than X-rays.

The Catheters: We typically place three or four multipolar catheters.

High Right Atrium (HRA): Acts as the "sinus node" surrogate.

His Bundle (HIS): The crucial lighthouse. It sits on the tricuspid annulus and records the electrical bridge between the atria and ventricles.

Coronary Sinus (CS): A catheter snake that slips behind the left atrium, giving us a view of the left side of the heart without actually entering it.

Right Ventricle (RV): A backup safety net and a pacing site.

1.2 The Basic Intervals When the catheters are in place, we measure time in milliseconds (ms).

The AH Interval: This represents the conduction time through the AV node. Think of the AV node as a toll booth designed to slow traffic. If the AH is short (<60ms), the toll gate is broken (fast conduction). If it's long (>125ms), the gate is sticky (slow conduction).

The HV Interval: This is the time from the His bundle to the ventricular muscle. This is the "speed limit" on the highway. A prolonged HV interval (>55ms) whispers a warning: this patient is at risk of complete heart block.

1.3 Pacing Maneuvers: Stressing the System We do not just watch; we provoke. You will learn to perform Decremental Pacing. This involves pacing the heart faster and faster until the AV node gives up (the Wenckebach point). It's a stress test for the electrical system. If the AV node conducts 1:1 at 250 beats per minute, that's abnormal—it suggests a "fast lane" or bypass tract exists that shouldn't be there.

Chapter 2: Supraventricular Tachycardia (SVT) – The Independent Competencies

As a trainee, you must be able to cure SVT independently. In 2026, we categorize these largely into two buckets: the "short circuits" inside the AV node (AVNRT) and the "extra wires" connecting atria and ventricles (AVRT).

2.1 AVNRT: Taming the Slow Pathway

Atrioventricular Nodal Reentrant Tachycardia (AVNRT) is the most common SVT you will encounter. Imagine a roundabout with two entrances: a Fast Pathway and a Slow Pathway. In AVNRT, the electricity gets stuck spinning around this roundabout endlessly.

The Strategy: The Slow Pathway Modification We do not touch the Fast Pathway (that would cause heart block and require a pacemaker). Instead, we target the Slow Pathway.

The Triangle of Koch: You must memorize this anatomy. It is bounded by the Coronary Sinus os, the Tricuspid Annulus, and the Tendon of Todaro.

The Procedure: Using a mapping catheter, we hunt for a specific electrical signature—a fragmented, low-voltage signal near the CS os.

The "Junctional" Rhythm: This is the sweetest sound in the lab. When we apply energy (RF or Cryo), the heart often responds with a "junctional rhythm"—a steady, automatic beat. This confirms we are heating the right spot. It is a moment of high tension; if the rhythm becomes too fast, we must stop immediately to prevent heart block.

2.2 Accessory Pathways (WPW & AVRT)

Wolff-Parkinson-White (WPW) syndrome involves a physical bridge of muscle (bundle of Kent) that bypasses the AV node.

The 2026 Approach:

Mapping: We use the CS catheter to see which part of the heart activates earliest. If the left side activates before the His bundle, the pathway is on the left (Left Lateral Pathway).

Orthodromic vs. Antidromic:

Orthodromic (95%): Electricity goes down the normal AV node and up the accessory pathway. The QRS is narrow.

Antidromic (5%): Electricity goes down the accessory pathway. The QRS is wide and looks terrifyingly like Ventricular Tachycardia (VT).

Ablation: Unlike AVNRT, we often perform Retrograde Aortic Access for left-sided pathways. You will learn to cross the aortic valve carefully, curling the catheter back under the mitral valve to burn the pathway from the ventricular side.

Chapter 3: Atrial Flutter – The "Macro" Re-entry

Typical Atrial Flutter is less like a small roundabout and more like a race track around the tricuspid valve. The electricity flows in a large counter-clockwise loop.

3.1 The CTI Line (Cavotricuspid Isthmus) The treatment is elegant in its simplicity but demanding in its execution. We must draw a "line in the sand" across the isthmus—the narrow strip of tissue between the IVC (Inferior Vena Cava) and the Tricuspid Valve.

3.2 Validating the Block Burning the line is easy; proving it works is the skill.

Differential Pacing: Once the line is created, we pace from the coronary sinus. The electricity should no longer be able to "jump" across the isthmus. It should be forced to go all the way around the atrium to reach the other side. This delay confirms Bidirectional Block. If you don't confirm block, the flutter will come back.

Chapter 4: Atrial Fibrillation (AF) – The 2026 Revolution

This is where the curriculum has changed the most. In 2020, AF ablation was considered "complex." In 2026, Pulmonary Vein Isolation (PVI) is a core competency.

4.1 The Mechanism: AF is triggered by chaotic sparks, usually originating from the muscle sleeves inside the pulmonary veins. Our goal is to electrically quarantine these veins—to build a fence around them so the sparks cannot reach the rest of the heart.

4.2 The Technology Shift: Enter PFA (Pulsed Field Ablation) For decades, we used heat (Radiofrequency) or cold (Cryo). Both had a risk: collateral damage. The esophagus runs right behind the heart; burn too deep, and you cause a fatal fistula.

In 2026, Pulsed Field Ablation is the gold standard you will learn.

How it works: PFA delivers ultra-short, high-voltage electrical pulses (nanoseconds). This creates microscopic pores in the cell membranes (electroporation).

Tissue Specificity: This is the "magic" of PFA. Heart muscle cells have a specific threshold for this damage. Nerves and the esophagus have a much higher threshold. Therefore, we can isolate the veins rapidly without fearing esophageal injury.

The Workflow: You will advance a "flower" or "basket" shaped catheter into the vein, verify contact, and deliver the pulse. A 2-second delivery replaces what used to be a 30-minute point-by-point burn.

Chapter 5: Complex Ablation & Ventricular Arrhythmias (Supervised)

While you must master SVT and AF, the curriculum asks for exposure and supervised practice in the deep waters of Ventricular Tachycardia (VT).

5.1 Electro-Anatomical Mapping (EAM) You cannot treat complex VT without high-density mapping. Systems like CARTO, Rhythmia, or EnSite X allow us to collect thousands of electrical points in minutes.

Voltage Mapping: Healthy muscle has high voltage (>1.5 mV). Scar tissue (from a previous heart attack) has low voltage (<0.5 mV).

The Border Zone: VT lives in the "grey zone"—the border between dead scar and healthy tissue. This is where the slow-conducting channels hide.

5.2 Ablation Strategy: Substrate Modification We do not just chase the rhythm; we hunt the "substrate."

LAVA (Local Abnormal Ventricular Activities): In sinus rhythm, we look for these tiny, fractionated signals inside the scar. They represent surviving fibers that can sustain a short circuit.

The Goal: We "homogenize" the scar—burning these surviving channels to ensure electricity can no longer travel through the bad neighborhood.

Chapter 6: Safety, Ethics, and The Human Element

Technical skill without judgment is dangerous. The 2026 curriculum places heavy emphasis on Human Factors.

6.1 Complications You must be able to manage the "Big Three" independent of your consultant:

Tamponade: If you poke a hole in the heart, blood fills the pericardial sac. BP drops. You must recognize this on the screen immediately (loss of heart border movement) and be ready to drain it (pericardiocentesis).

Vascular Access: With large sheaths for PFA, the femoral vein is vulnerable. Ultrasound-guided access is mandatory.

Stroke: We use heavy anticoagulation (Heparin) during the case to prevent clots from forming on the plastic catheters.

6.2 The Ethics of Ablation Just because we can ablate, doesn't mean we should. In 2026, we focus on "Holistic Rhythm Management." If a patient has a BMI of 40 and untreated sleep apnea, ablating their AF is like bailing water out of a sinking boat without plugging the hole. You must be brave enough to tell a patient: "No procedure until we fix the lifestyle factors."

Part 1: Implantable Cardioverter Defibrillators (ICDs)

The Evolution of Protection

For decades, the Transvenous ICD (TV-ICD) was the gold standard. It involves placing a lead through the vein, across the tricuspid valve, and into the right ventricle. It is effective, but it has an "Achilles' heel": the lead itself. Leads can fracture. They can cause infection. They can damage the tricuspid valve.

As of 2026, we have two major alternatives that avoid the heart's interior.

1. Subcutaneous ICD (S-ICD)

Think of the S-ICD as a "jacket" for the heart rather than an implant inside it. The lead sits under the skin, completely outside the thoracic cage.

Best for: Younger patients who do not need pacing.

Limitation: It cannot pace the heart painlessly. If the patient has a slow heart rate (bradycardia), this device is usually not the right choice.

2026 Update: Newer algorithms have reduced "oversensing" (where the device mistakes muscle movement for a dangerous rhythm), making shocks less likely to happen by accident.

2. Extravascular ICD (EV-ICD)

This is the new player that has gained traction in the UK over the last two years. The EV-ICD (such as the Aurora system) is a hybrid. The lead is placed under the breastbone (substernal) but outside the heart.

Why it matters: Because the lead is closer to the heart than in an S-ICD, it requires less energy to shock the heart.

The "Killer App": Unlike the S-ICD, the EV-ICD can pace the heart. It can deliver Anti-Tachycardia Pacing (ATP). This means it can silently speed up the heart to stop a dangerous rhythm without needing to deliver a painful shock.

Implantation Skill: This requires a new technique. You do not access a vein. Instead, you make a small incision near the bottom of the breastbone and tunnel the lead underneath it.

Part 2: Cardiac Resynchronization Therapy (CRT) Retuning the Engine

Heart failure often causes the heart walls to beat out of sync. One wall contracts while the other is still relaxing. This is like an engine firing on the wrong cylinders. CRT is the mechanic that retunes the timing.
Traditional Biventricular Pacing (BiV)

This has been the standard for 20 years. You place one lead in the right ventricle and another lead in a vein on the outside of the left ventricle (the coronary sinus). When both pace together, the heart squeezes in sync.

The Problem: It doesn't work for everyone. About 30% of patients are "non-responders." Their hearts just don't improve.

The 2026 Standard: Conduction System Pacing (CSP)

This is the most significant change in your curriculum. Instead of bypassing the heart's natural wiring, we now hijack it. We plug directly into the heart's "fibre optic" network.
1. His-Bundle Pacing (HBP)

This was the first form of CSP. We pace the Bundle of His.

Pros: It produces a perfectly narrow, natural heartbeat.

Cons: The Bundle of His is tiny and surrounded by fibrous tissue. Sensing the heartbeat is difficult, and battery life is often short because it takes high energy to capture the nerve.

2. Left Bundle Branch Area Pacing (LBBAP)

In 2026, LBBAP has largely overtaken His-Bundle pacing in UK practice.

Technique: You screw the lead deep into the interventricular septum (the wall between the chambers). You aim to capture the Left Bundle Branch on the other side.

Why it wins: It is easier to do than His-Bundle pacing. The sensing is better. The thresholds (energy needed) are lower, so batteries last longer.

Coursework Note: You must learn to read the EGM (electrocardiogram) signals during implantation. You are looking for a specific "w" pattern to turn into a "qr" pattern, indicating you have captured the conduction system.

Part 3: Leadless Pacing
The Wireless Revolution

Imagine a pacemaker the size of a vitamin capsule. No wires. No pocket under the skin. It sits entirely inside the heart.
Single Chamber Leadless (Micra / Aveir)

These are now routine for patients with atrial fibrillation or those who only need occasional pacing.

Procedure: A large catheter is inserted into the femoral vein (leg). The device is steered into the right ventricle and deployed. Tines (little hooks) or a screw hold it in place.

Safety: The risk of infection is near zero because there is no surgical pocket.

Dual Chamber Leadless Pacing

This is the frontier. As of early 2026, NICE (National Institute for Health and Care Excellence) guidelines are cautious.

Technology: Two capsules are implanted—one in the atrium, one in the ventricle. They talk to each other wirelessly through the blood (conductive communication).

Current Status: While technically available, widespread NHS funding is still limited to specialist centres or specific high-risk patients (e.g., those with blocked veins or history of severe infection). The durability of two separate batteries is still being monitored in long-term registry data.

Part 4: Complications and Lead Extraction

The Risk Manager

Implanting devices is only half the job. Managing them when things go wrong is the other half. The most feared complication is infection.

Indications for Extraction

When must a lead come out?

Systemic Infection: If bacteria are in the blood (bacteraemia) or on the valve (endocarditis), the entire system must go. Antibiotics alone will not sterilize a device.

Pocket Infection: Even if it looks like just a local abscess, it is effectively a system infection. Do not just treat the skin.

Lead Failure: If a lead breaks (fractures) in a young patient, we often extract it rather than abandoning it, to prevent "vascular crowding" (too many wires in the vein).

Transvenous Lead Extraction (TLE)

This is high-risk. Over time, leads scar into the vein walls. Pulling them can tear the Superior Vena Cava (SVC), causing fatal bleeding.

The Toolkit:

Mechanical Sheaths: These are tubes with rotating blades at the tip that cut through the scar tissue.

Laser Sheaths: These use cool ultraviolet laser pulses to vaporize the scar tissue holding the lead.

The Hybrid Approach: In 2026, we use a "risk stratification" approach. If the lead has been in for more than 10 years, or if the patient is female (veins are smaller), we prepare for a complex extraction with a cardiac surgeon on standby.

Section 1: The Structure and Function of the Modern Arrhythmia MDT (2026)

The Arrhythmia MDT in 2026 is distinct from the general cardiology meetings of the past. It is a precision-medicine forum. As the lead, you must ensure the attendance and active participation of a diverse group of specialists. The days of a solitary electrophysiologist making decisions are over.

Core Composition of the MDT:

Electrophysiologists (Lead): To assess technical feasibility of ablation.

Complex Device Specialists: To manage CRT-D optimization and lead extraction risk.

Imaging Cardiologists: Crucial for defining scar burden via Cardiac MRI (CMR) or CT-integration for ablation planning.

Clinical Geneticists / Genetic Counsellors: Now mandatory for all ICC discussions.

Heart Failure Specialists: To determine if the arrhythmia is a cause or consequence of decomposation.

Paediatric/ACHD Representatives: For transition clinics (familial substrates often bridge these ages).

Operational Dynamics: In 2026, AI-driven tools are often used to pre-screen Holter data and 12-lead ECGs before the meeting. Your role as the lead is to synthesize this data. You must foster an environment of "psychological safety" where a genetic counsellor can challenge a consultant electrophysiologist regarding the utility of a test.

Leadership Note: The curriculum demands you demonstrate synthesis. When a case of VT storm is presented, you do not just ask "What do we do?" You summarize: "This is a 65-year-old with ischemic cardiomyopathy. The VANISH2 data suggests ablation is superior to escalating sotalol here, but the MRI shows an apical thrombus. How do we mitigate the stroke risk during the procedure?"

Section 2: Managing Complex Cases – Ventricular Tachycardia (VT)

The most challenging decision you will face as the MDT lead is the choice between Anti-Arrhythmic Drugs (AADs) and Catheter Ablation for ventricular tachycardia. This debate has been settled significantly by evidence emerging in 2024 and 2025.

The Paradigm Shift: Ablation as First-Line Therapy

Historically, ablation was a "bailout" for patients who failed amiodarone. By 2026, this is considered outdated practice for Ischemic Cardiomyopathy (ICM).

Evidence-Based Decision Making (The VANISH2 Context): The publication of the VANISH2 trial results in 2025 provided the evidence base we had been waiting for. It demonstrated that in patients with prior myocardial infarction and VT, first-line catheter ablation was superior to AADs (specifically sotalol) in reducing the composite endpoint of death, VT storm, and appropriate ICD shocks.

When to favor Ablation:

Ischemic Substrate: Well-defined scars are excellent targets.

Slow VT: Hemodynamically tolerated VT allows for detailed activation mapping, ensuring higher success rates.

Avoidance of Toxicities: Young patients who face decades of potential amiodarone toxicity (thyroid, lung, liver) should be prioritized for ablation.

Recurrent Shocks: "Shock anxiety" is a potent destroyer of quality of life. Ablation offers the best chance of shock freedom.

When to favor Anti-Arrhythmic Drugs (AADs):

Non-Ischemic Dilated Cardiomyopathy (DCM): The substrate here is often mid-myocardial or epicardial and diffuse. Ablation is harder and has lower success rates than in ischemic disease. Here, Amiodarone or Mexiletine often remains the primary stabilizer.

Polymorphic VT / VF: These are usually driven by acute ischemia or channelopathies, not a fixed scar circuit. Ablation is rarely useful unless a specific "trigger" PVC is identified.

Frail / Comorbid Patients: If a patient cannot tolerate a 4-hour general anaesthetic or the fluid load of an irrigated catheter, drugs are the safer, pragmatic choice.

Advanced Therapies for "Refractory" Cases

As the MDT lead, you must also know what to do when both drugs and standard ablation fail.

Stereotactic Arrhythmia Radioablation (STAR): By 2026, non-invasive radiotherapy (borrowed from oncology) has become a viable compassionate use option for deep septal substrates that catheters cannot reach.

Autonomic Modulation: Bilateral cardiac sympathetic denervation (sympathectomy) is increasingly discussed in the MDT for electrical storm refractory to all other measures.

Section 3: Inherited Cardiac Conditions (ICC) – The Service Lead Role

Leading the ICC arm of the service is arguably more complex than the VT section because you are treating families, not just individuals. The 2026 curriculum emphasizes "Mainstreaming Genomics". This means the cardiologist—not just the geneticist—must be competent in ordering and interpreting genetic panels.

Risk Stratification in ICC

You are responsible for ensuring that every patient with a condition like Hypertrophic Cardiomyopathy (HCM) or Long QT Syndrome (LQTS) is risk-stratified for Sudden Cardiac Death (SCD).

The Dynamic Risk Score: We no longer rely on a single "snapshot" risk assessment. Risk is dynamic.

HCM: We use the HCM Risk-SCD calculator, but in 2026, this is heavily supplemented by CMR tissue characterization. A patient with a low clinical risk score but >15% Late Gadolinium Enhancement (scar) on MRI is now often considered for an ICD in our MDT discussions.

Arrhythmogenic Cardiomyopathy (ACM/ARVC): The "Padua Criteria" and newer 2025 refined scores are used. Genetic status matters: a Desmoplakin (DSP) mutation carries a higher risk of left-ventricular arrhythmias than a Plakophilin (PKP2) mutation. As the lead, you must highlight this genotype-phenotype correlation.

Coordinating Genetic Testing

The UK Genomic Medicine Service (GMS) has standardized test directories. Your role is to police the "Strict Necessity Test" for ordering these expensive investigations.

Diagnostic Testing (The Proband): We only test the person with the disease (the proband). We do not "fish" for genes in healthy relatives unless a mutation is identified in the affected person.

Example: A 30-year-old man presents with unexplained cardiac arrest. The MDT reviews his phenotype. If the ECG suggests Brugada Syndrome, we order the specific channelopathy panel (R543 code in the UK directory). We do not order a pan-cardiology panel which yields confusing "Variants of Uncertain Significance" (VUS).

Predictive (Cascade) Testing: Once a "Pathogenic" or "Likely Pathogenic" variant is found, the MDT coordinator (often a genetic nurse) initiates cascade screening. This is the testing of first-degree relatives.

The "Ghent" Approach: We must ensure relatives are counselled before testing. A positive test in a sister means she has the risk; a negative test means she can be discharged from the clinic forever. This is high-stakes medicine.

Shutterstock

Explore

Section 4: The Challenge of the VUS (Variant of Uncertain Significance)

A major specific learning outcome for 2026 is the management of the VUS. This is where the MDT adds the most value.

The Scenario: You order a gene panel for a patient with Dilated Cardiomyopathy. The report comes back: Titin (TTN) variant – Variant of Uncertain Significance.

The MDT Lead's Duty: You must prevent "genetic misinterpretation."

Do NOT use a VUS to drive cascade screening in the family. If you test the patient's children for a VUS, you create anxiety without medical validity.

Segregation Analysis: The MDT may decide to test the patient's parents. If the affected father has the variant, but the unaffected elderly mother also has it, the variant is likely benign. This "segregation" transforms the VUS into "Benign," saving the family from decades of worry.

Polygenic Risk Scores (PRS): New to the 2026 workflow is the integration of PRS. For conditions like coronary artery disease or subtle phenotype HCM, a high polygenic risk score might tip the balance toward more aggressive lipid management or earlier surveillance, even if a monogenic "single gene" cause isn't found.

Section 5: Governance, Safety, and Quality Control

Finally, leading the service requires audit and governance. You are the safety officer.

Complication Tracking: Every tamponade, every stroke, and every vascular injury from the EP lab must be discussed in the MDT—not to blame, but to learn.

The "MDT Outcome" Form: In 2026, electronic health records (EHR) require a mandatory "MDT Outcome" field. You must ensure this is clear.

Bad Outcome Note: "Discussed. Review in clinic."

Good Outcome Note: "MDT Decision: Offer ablation for VT. Risks of stroke (2%) and groin hematoma (3%) discussed. If patient declines, second line is Amiodarone. Genetic testing approved for R132 panel."

Section 1: Governance of Radiation Protection

In the UK, radiation safety is not merely a "box-ticking" exercise; it is a rigid legal framework enforced by the Health and Safety Executive (HSE) and the Care Quality

Commission (CQC). As a leader in the EP lab, you must transition from simply wearing lead to managing the policy that dictates it.

1.1 The Legal Backbone: IR(ME)R and IRR

You must distinguish between the two governing regulations. In 2026, these remain the twin pillars of safety:

IRR17 (Ionising Radiations Regulations 2017): This protects staff and the public. It focuses on dose limits, equipment maintenance, and the physical environment.

IR(ME)R (Ionising Radiation (Medical Exposure) Regulations): This protects the patient. It focuses on justification, optimization, and clinical responsibility.

1.2 The Role of the Radiation Protection Supervisor (RPS)

In many EP departments, the lead EP consultant acts as the RPS. This is a statutory role. It is not enough to just be "good at fluoroscopy."

The RPS is the "boots on the ground" officer who ensures local rules are followed.

The "Local Rules": These are the specific, written protocols for your lab. As a leader, you must ensure these are not dusty documents in a drawer but living protocols. For example, who is allowed to press the pedal? In 2026, with the rise of non-medical practitioners, does your local rule explicitly allow a specialized physiologist to operate the fluoroscopy pedal? If not, they are breaking the law.

Dose Constraints vs. Dose Limits: You must govern the monitoring of staff. The legal limit for effective dose is 20 mSv per year, but most NHS Trusts set a "investigation level" much lower (often 1-6 mSv).

Investigation of Incidents: If a junior fellow steps on the pedal while the C-arm is screened over their own hand, or if a patient receives a skin dose >3Gy (a "trigger level" for potential skin injury), you, as the governance lead, must trigger a formal investigation.

1.3 Optimization and "The Culture of Less"

Leadership is setting the tone. If the consultant is careless with collimation, the trainee will be too.

Governance Action: You must implement regular audits of Dose Area Product (DAP) per procedure.

Example: A governance lead might review the last 50 AF ablations. If Consultant A averages 500 $cGycm^2$ and Consultant B averages 2,000 $cGycm^2$ for the same workflow, this is a governance issue. It requires a quiet, documented conversation about framing rates, collimation, and use of 3D mapping systems to reduce screening.

Section 2: The Human Factor – Supervision and Team Dynamics

The EP lab is a high-stakes environment similar to an aviation cockpit. The "Captain" (Consultant) is responsible for the ship, but the safety of the journey depends on the co-pilots (Fellows) and the navigators (Physiologists).
2.1 Governing the Physiologist Workforce

In the UK EP landscape of 2026, Cardiac Physiologists (or Cardiac Scientists) are no longer just "techs." They are independent practitioners. Many hold BHRS (British Heart

Rhythm Society) or IBHRE accreditation and perform complex tasks autonomously.

Scope of Practice: Governance requires a clear definition of what physiologists can do.

Can they perform transseptal puncture? (Rare, but possible in advanced roles).

Can they reveal the loop recorder results to a patient? (Yes, standard practice).

Can they discharge a patient?

The Governance Trap: The most common failure in this area is "assumption of competence." A leader assumes the physiologist knows how to troubleshoot a specific analyser.

The Solution: A rigorous competency matrix. You must ensure that every physiologist in the lab has a "signed-off" logbook for the specific equipment you use. If you buy a new cryo-ablation console, you cannot assume staff know it. You must organize vendor training and document it. This is verifiable governance.

2.2 Supervision of Junior Doctors (The 2026 Context)

Training in the UK is currently navigating the fallout of the "Shape of Training" reforms. In 2025, the British Junior Cardiologists' Association (BJCA) highlighted a crisis: trainees are finishing with fewer procedural numbers because they spend more time in General Internal Medicine (GIM).

As a lab leader, you are the guardian of their training quality.

The "Cockpit" Hierarchy: You must cultivate a "flattened hierarchy" for safety. A junior doctor must feel empowered to say, “Boss, the ACT (Activated Clotting Time) is only 220, should we wait before ablation?" If they are too scared to speak, your governance has failed.

Allocating "Fail-Safe" Procedures: Governance involves patient selection. You do not give a trainee their first AF ablation on a patient with a massive left atrium and heart failure. You assign them the "textbook" case. This protects the patient and the trainee's confidence.

Verifiable Training: Use the DOPS (Direct Observation of Procedural Skills) assessments on the ePortfolio not just as admin, but as a real governance tool. If a trainee is struggling, document it early. "Nice" consultants who pass everyone are dangerous leaders.

Section 3: Governance of Device Follow-Up Clinics

The pacing clinic is the "unsung" engine room of the department. It is high-volume, high-risk, and often under-resourced.

3.1 Staffing Ratios and BHRS Standards

Governance is about ensuring you are not running a "sweatshop." The British Heart Rhythm Society (BHRS) Standards (updated Jan 2024 and still the benchmark in 2026) provide the metrics you must fight for:

The "Two-Person" Rule: Standards generally dictate that complex device checks (ICD/CRT) should have appropriate support. While physiologists often lead these, a consultant must be accessible.

Volume Metrics: An implanting centre must maintain minimum volumes (e.g., >80 new implants per year) to remain safe. If your centre's numbers drop, you (as the governance lead) must flag this to the Medical Director. It is unethical to dabble in devices; you either do them well, or you refer them elsewhere.

3.2 Data Integrity and the "Lost to Follow-up" Risk

The greatest governance nightmare in a device service is the patient who "falls through the cracks."

Scenario: A patient with an ICD moves house, misses an appointment, and the letter goes to the wrong GP. Three years later, their battery depletes, and they suffer an arrest.

Governance Solution: You need a fail-safe database. Whether it is "CVIS" or a proprietary system, you must have a query that runs every month: "Show me all patients who have not had a device interrogation in >12 months." This list is your safety net.

Section 4: Remote Monitoring (RM) – The New Frontier

By 2026, Remote Monitoring is no longer an "add-on"; it is the standard of care. However, it has created a governance crisis known as "Alert Fatigue."

4.1 The Data Flood

Modern CIEDs (Cardiac Implantable Electronic Devices) transmit terabytes of data. They send alerts for AF episodes, lead impedance changes, and battery drops.

The Governance Challenge: If a device sends a "red alert" (e.g., a lead fracture) on a Saturday night, and no one looks at it until Monday morning, is the Trust liable?

The 2026 Approach: You must have a robust SOP (Standard Operating Procedure) for RM.

Define "Working Hours": Your policy must explicitly state to patients: "This is NOT an emergency service. We review alerts Mon-Fri, 9-5." This protects the hospital from liability for weekend events.

Triage Protocols: Who sees the red alert first? Usually, a Band 7 Physiologist. When do they escalate to a Consultant? You need a flowchart.

4.2 AI and Actionable Alerts

In 2026, we are seeing the integration of AI-driven filtering to manage this workload (as discussed in the September 2025 BHRS webinars).

Governance of AI: If you use software to filter out "noise" (false positive AF), you must be sure it isn't filtering out real pathology. You need to audit the AI's decisions periodically.

Reimbursement and Job Planning: A common leadership failure is failing to allocate time for RM. A consultant job plan that has 0 PAs (Programmed Activities) for remote monitoring is a governance risk. You cannot review 500 virtual transmissions in your lunch break. You must negotiate this time into your contract.

Advanced Theme: Leading an ACHD Service

Section 12.1: Management of Complex Congenital Anatomy

In the acquired heart disease world, heart failure usually looks the same: a weak left ventricle. In ACHD, heart failure comes in many shapes. It might be a blue patient with a single ventricle, or a pink patient with a right ventricle doing a left ventricle's job.

1. The Univentricular Heart: The Fontan Circulation

The Fontan circulation is perhaps the most fragile miracle in medicine. It connects the systemic veins directly to the pulmonary arteries. There is no pump pushing blood to the lungs. Blood flows passively, driven only by central venous pressure and the "sucking" action of breathing.

The 2026 Perspective: By 2026, we treat the Fontan not just as a heart defect, but as a specific circulatory syndrome.

The "Failing Fontan": This is the nightmare scenario. It doesn't always look like typical heart failure. It often presents as Protein Losing Enteropathy (PLE) or Plastic Bronchitis (coughing up casts).

Liver Disease (FALD): Every Fontan patient has a congested liver. By the time they reach adulthood, liver fibrosis is almost guaranteed. In 2026, we don't wait for enzymes to rise. We use elastography and advanced MRI screening annually.

Management Shifts:

Medical Therapy: We are aggressive. Pulmonary vasodilators (like bosentan or sildenafil) are commonly used to lower lung resistance, helping that passive blood flow.

The Lymphatic Revolution: We now understand that the lymphatic system gets overwhelmed in Fontan patients. New interventional procedures to map and embolize leaking lymphatics are now standard in tertiary centers.

Arrhythmia: A fast heart rate is deadly here. It kills the passive flow. You must have a low threshold for cardioversion.

Clinical Pearl: If a Fontan patient looks "well" but has a rising haemoglobin (becoming more polycythaemic) or dropping albumin, they are failing. Do not wait for oedema.

2. Transposition of the Great Arteries (TGA)

You will see two distinct populations in your clinic. The "Old Guard" (Mustard/Senning repairs) and the "New Wave" (Arterial Switch).

The Atrial Switch (Mustard/Senning): These patients, mostly in their 40s and 50s now, have a Systemic Right Ventricle. Their anatomy was "switched" at the atrial level.

The Problem: The Right Ventricle (RV) is designed to pump at low pressure. In these patients, it has been pumping at high (systemic) pressure for decades. It eventually gets tired.

Baffle Issues: The tunnels (baffles) created inside the atria can leak or narrow. A narrowed superior baffle causes "SVC syndrome" (swollen face). A leak acts like an ASD, causing desaturation.

The Rhythm Timebomb: The extensive atrial surgery kills the sinus node. Most of these patients need pacemakers. But be careful—threading leads through those complex baffles is a minefield.

The Arterial Switch (ASO): These patients look anatomically "normal" now because the arteries were switched back. However:

The Coronaries: The coronary arteries were moved during surgery. Kinking or stenosis can cause silent ischaemia.

The Neo-Aortic Root: The "new" aorta often dilates over time. We watch them like hawks for aneurysms.

3. Tetralogy of Fallot (ToF)

This is the most common complex lesion you will see. They were "repaired" in childhood, often with a patch that disrupted the pulmonary valve.

The Sequel: The price of the repair is Pulmonary Regurgitation (PR). Blood leaks back into the RV with every beat. For 20 years, the RV tolerates this. It dilates, it stretches, it scarps. Then, it fails.

The 2026 Debate: Timing of Pulmonary Valve Replacement (PVR) When do we put a new valve in?

Too early: The new valve wears out, and they need another procedure.

Too late: The RV is irreversibly damaged, and the patient remains symptomatic forever.

In 2026, we use CMR (Cardiovascular Magnetic Resonance) data religiously. We look for the "tipping point." We don't just measure volumes (e.g., RVEDVi > 150 ml/m^2); we look at fibrosis and RV ejection fraction. The trend is moving toward earlier intervention, often using Transcatheter Pulmonary Valve Implantation (TPVI) to avoid opening the chest again.

Section 12.2: The ACHD Multidisciplinary Team (MDT)

You cannot be a "lone wolf" in ACHD. The physiology is too weird, and the risks are too high. Leading the MDT is a core curriculum requirement.

The Orchestra of Experts

In a typical Level 1 ACHD Center MDT meeting in 2026, the room (or Zoom call) is crowded.

The Congenital Surgeon: They think in 3D geometry. They tell you if a valve can be replaced without damaging a coronary artery.

The Imaging Specialist: They are the eyes. They bring the 4D Flow MRI data that shows us exactly how blood is swirling in a dilated aorta.

The Electrophysiologist (EP): ACHD hearts are scarred hearts. Scar tissue breeds short circuits (VT/atrial flutter). The EP doctor plans the ablation or ICD.

The Obstetrician: This is crucial. More women with complex hearts are reaching childbearing age. Pregnancy adds a 50% volume load to the heart. For a failing Fontan or a dilated aorta, this can be fatal. The MDT decides if pregnancy is safe, or how to manage the high-risk delivery.

Leading the Decision: Re-intervention

Let's look at a classic MDT dilemma: The ToF patient needing a new valve.

The Scenario: A 32-year-old male with repaired Fallot. He feels fine. He plays 5-a-side football.

The Data: MRI shows his RV is huge (160ml/m²). There is severe pulmonary regurgitation.

The Conflict: The patient says, "I feel great, why operate?" The guidelines say, "The RV is about to crack."

The MDT Role:

The Surgeon might say, "I can do a valve sparing repair now, but if we wait, he'll need a transplant later."

The Imager says, "There is no fibrosis yet. We have a window."

The Psychologist (yes, they are in the MDT too) says, "He is terrified of surgery because he remembers the pain from childhood."

Your Role as Leader: You synthesize this. You don't just read the guidelines. You acknowledge the patient's fear (validating the psychologist), you respect the anatomy (the surgeon), and you use the data (the imager). You formulate a plan: We will exercise test him (CPET). If his VO2 max is dropping, we push for surgery. We offer peer support to help his anxiety.

Conclusion: The Future is Personal

By 2026, the management of ACHD has moved beyond "general rules" to "precision medicine." We don't just treat "Tetralogy of Fallot"; we treat this specific patient's Fallot, with their specific scar burden, their specific genetic profile, and their specific life goals.

The anatomy is complex, but the goal is simple: to give these patients not just a longer life, but a life worth living. They have fought hard to be here. Your job is to ensure their heart can keep up with their dreams.

Quick Reference: 2026 Management Matrix

Lesion	Key Long-Term Issue	Diagnostic Gold Standard	Key Management Move (2026)
Fontan	Liver Fibrosis & PLE	MRI Liver Elastography	Early lymphatic intervention; Pulmonary vasodilators.
Mustard/Senning	Systemic RV Failure	CMR (myocardial strain)	SGLT2 Inhibitors; early referral for transplant assessment.
Tetralogy of Fallot	Pulmonary Regurgitation	CMR (Volumes + Flow)	TPVI (Transcatheter valve) before irreversible RV damage.
Arterial Switch	Coronary Stenosis	CT Coronary Angiogram	Aggressive ischemia screening; stenting if feasible.

12.3 Advanced Complications: Heart Failure and Pulmonary Hypertension

The Unique Nature of ACHD Heart Failure

Heart failure in the general population is often a story of ischemic damage or age-related stiffening. In ACHD, it is fundamentally different. It is a story of geometry and adaptation.

Imagine asking an engine designed for a small hatchback to power a heavy truck. That is effectively what happens in patients with a Systemic Right Ventricle (RV)—such as those with Transposition of the Great Arteries (TGA) post-Mustard/Senning repair, or Congenitally Corrected TGA (ccTGA).

The RV has a thin wall and a crescent shape, designed for low-pressure pumping to the lungs. When forced to pump at high systemic pressures for 30 or 40 years, it doesn't just fail; it changes shape. It becomes spherical, drags the tricuspid valve apart (causing regurgitation), and eventually fibroses.

Key Clinical Insight (2026 Perspective): By 2026, we have moved away from treating systemic RV failure exactly like Left Ventricular (LV) failure. While ACE inhibitors and Beta-blockers remain the baseline, the 2025 Guidelines have solidified the role of SGLT2 inhibitors (e.g., Dapagliflozin, Empagliflozin) in this population. These drugs, originally for diabetes, have shown remarkable efficacy in reducing hospitalizations even in the complex geometries of ACHD.
Pulmonary Hypertension (PH): The Silent Threat

PH in ACHD is not a single disease. It is a spectrum. Understanding the type of PH is the difference between a successful treatment and a fatal error.

We generally categorize ACHD-PH into two buckets:

Pre-capillary PH: This is often the legacy of unclosed shunts (ASD, VSD) leading to vascular remodeling. In its most severe form, this is Eisenmenger Syndrome—where the pressure in the lungs exceeds the body's systemic pressure, reversing the shunt and causing cyanosis.

Post-capillary PH: This is caused by "back pressure" from a failing left heart or a stiff systemic ventricle.

The "treat and repair" trap: A common pitfall for trainees is seeing a hole (ASD) and high pressures, and wanting to close the hole. Stop. If you close a shunt in a patient with established Eisenmenger physiology, you remove their "pop-off" valve. The right heart will fail instantly against the high resistance, leading to catastrophe.

Advanced PH Therapies: The Modern Arsenal

For decades, our options were limited. Now, the toolkit is robust. The goal is to lower pulmonary vascular resistance (PVR) without collapsing the systemic blood pressure.

Endothelin Receptor Antagonists (ERAs): Drugs like Bosentan, Ambrisentan, and Macitentan work by blocking the "constriction" signals in the vessel walls. In 2026, these are standard of care for Eisenmenger patients to improve exercise capacity.

PDE-5 Inhibitors: Sildenafil and Tadalafil. These are the "dilators." They are often used in combination with ERAs for a synergistic effect.

Prostacyclins: For the sickest patients, we use inhaled or intravenous prostacyclins (e.g., Epoprostenol, Treprostinil).

The Game Changer - Sotatercept: Approved broadly around 2024, this activin signaling inhibitor represents a new class of therapy. Unlike previous drugs that just dilated vessels, Sotatercept works to reverse the remodeling of the pulmonary arteries. In the ACHD population, early data suggests it can significantly improve functional class in patients who have plateaued on triple therapy.

The Road to Transplantation

When medical therapy is exhausted, we face the ultimate question: Transplantation.

In ACHD, a transplant is never "routine." These patients bring a unique set of surgical risks that you must be able to articulate to a patient or a transplant board:

The "Hostile Chest": Most of these patients have had 3, 4, or even 5 previous open-heart surgeries. The scar tissue is dense. The heart may be adhered to the back of the sternum. Opening the chest (sternotomy) carries a high risk of catastrophic bleeding before the surgery even begins.

HLA Sensitization (The Antibody Problem): Every previous surgery involved blood transfusions. Many involved homografts (human tissue valves). This exposure means the patient's immune system is "primed" to attack foreign tissue. They often have high levels of Panel Reactive Antibodies (PRA), making it incredibly difficult to find a donor heart that they won't reject immediately.

Anatomical Reconstruction: You cannot just sew a normal donor heart into an ACHD chest. The great vessels (aorta, pulmonary artery) may be in the wrong place, or the wrong size. The surgeon often has to reconstruct the venous baffles or pulmonary arteries extensively during the transplant.

12.4 Reproductive Health and Genetics

The High-Stakes of ACHD Pregnancy

Pregnancy is a massive hemodynamic stress test. By the second trimester, a woman's blood volume increases by 50%. Her cardiac output must rise to match. For a normal heart, this is a workout. For a complex ACHD heart, it can be a breaking point.

As an advanced trainee, you must move beyond general advice. You need to provide risk stratification. We use the mWHO (modified World Health Organization) classification:

mWHO I: Low risk (e.g., small ASD).

mWHO II/III: Moderate risk (e.g., Repaired Tetralogy of Fallot).

mWHO IV: Pregnancy Contraindicated.

The "Red Flag" Conditions (mWHO IV):

Severe Pulmonary Hypertension: Maternal mortality can be up to 30-50%. The inability to increase cardiac output through the stiff lungs leads to right heart failure.

Severe Systemic Ventricular Dysfunction: (LVEF < 30%).

Severe Left Heart Obstruction: (e.g., Severe Aortic Stenosis).

Specific Scenarios: Fontan and Cyanosis

1. The Fontan Circulation in Pregnancy: The Fontan circulation relies on passive flow to the lungs. It has no sub-pulmonary pump.

The Risk: The increased blood volume of pregnancy can overwhelm this passive system. This leads to massive fluid retention, ascites, and arrhythmias.

The Clotting Risk: Pregnancy is a hypercoagulable state. Fontan patients are already prone to clots. This combination is dangerous. We often require meticulous anticoagulation management, switching from Warfarin to LMWH (Low Molecular Weight Heparin) during the first trimester to avoid embryopathy, then carefully managing levels.

The Outcome: Miscarriage rates are high (up to 40%). Prematurity is common.

2. Cyanotic Heart Disease: In women who are cyanotic (low oxygen saturations), the fetus suffers.

Hypoxia: If the mother's resting saturation is <85%, the live birth rate drops to <12%. The fetus simply cannot get enough oxygen to grow.

Viscosity: The mother often has polycythemia (thick blood) to compensate for low oxygen. This increases the risk of placental thrombosis (clots in the placenta), leading to fetal growth restriction.

Genetics: The Question Every Parent Asks

"Will my baby have my heart condition?"

This is the most emotional question in the clinic. You must be able to answer it with compassion and accuracy.

The "Baseline" Risk: In the general population, the risk of Congenital Heart Disease (CHD) is about 0.8% to 1%.

The "Recurrence" Risk: If a parent has ACHD, the risk to the offspring generally rises to 3% to 5%.

It is higher if the mother is the affected parent (likely due to mitochondrial or cytoplasmic inheritance factors, or the uterine environment).

It is higher for specific lesions. For example, in Left Heart Obstruction lesions (Coarctation, Hypoplastic Left Heart), the recurrence risk can be 10-15%.

Genetic Syndromes (The 2026 Approach): We no longer just guess. Genetic screening is now routine. You must identify syndromic associations because they affect the child's entire life, not just their heart.

22q11.2 Deletion (DiGeorge Syndrome): Common in Tetralogy of Fallot and Truncus Arteriosus. 50% recurrence risk (Autosomal Dominant).

Marfan Syndrome (FBN1): Associated with aortic dilation. 50% recurrence risk.

Noonan Syndrome: Associated with Pulmonary Stenosis and Hypertrophic Cardiomyopathy.

Pre-Implantation Genetic Diagnosis (PGD): For patients with a known genetic mutation (e.g., Marfan), we can now offer IVF with PGD. This allows us to screen embryos before implantation to ensure the condition is not passed on. This is a complex ethical and logistical discussion, but it is a vital option to offer in a modern 2026 clinic.

Advanced Theme: Leading a Heart Failure Service

Part 1: Integrated Service Leadership (Subtopic 13.1)

1. The Ecosystem Approach: Beyond the Hospital Walls

The 2026 curriculum demands that the advanced trainee views the heart failure service not as a destination (the hospital) but as a flow. The historical fragmentation between secondary care (hospitals) and primary care (GPs) has been the greatest driver of readmissions. Your role is to build a "wall-less" hospital.

The "Hub and Spoke" Architecture In this model, the Tertiary Centre (the Hub) acts as the brain, while Community Units and Primary Care Networks (the Spokes) act as the hands.

The Hub (Tertiary Centre): Handles complex diagnostics (CMR, genetics), device implantation (CRT/ICD), and mechanical circulatory support. It does not hoard routine follow-up.

The Spoke (Community Hubs): These are now often located in the new "Neighbourhood Health Centres" mandated in 2025. They handle titration of "Quadruple Therapy" (ARNI/ACEi, Beta-blockers, MRA, SGLT2i) and routine biomarkers (NT-proBNP).

Operational Example: Consider the "Liverpool Model" (updated 2025). A patient in Chester (Spoke) with a complex device doesn't travel to the main hospital for a check. Instead, their device data is pushed via the HeartLogic algorithm to the Hub. If the algorithm detects "wet" lungs (fluid accumulation) weeks before symptoms appear, the Hub specialist messages the Spoke nurse to increase diuretics locally. The patient never leaves their borough.

2. The Ambulatory Heart Failure Unit (AHFU)

The AHFU is your most powerful tool to prevent admissions. In 2026, admitting a patient with decompensated heart failure for a 10-day bed stay is considered a failure of the outpatient system unless they require critical care.

Day Case Diuresis The modern AHFU operates a "Lounge" model. Patients identified as "wet" by community nurses or virtual monitoring are brought in for rapid intravenous (IV) diuretic loading and sent home the same day.

Protocol: Patients arrive at 08:00, receive high-dose IV furosemide, have electrolytes checked at 12:00, and are discharged at 16:00 with a plan.

The Metric: We measure success by "Bed Days Saved." A well-run AHFU can save 2,000 bed days annually per trust.

Clinical Scenario: Mrs. G, an 82-year-old with HFrEF (Heart Failure with reduced Ejection Fraction), calls the hotline reporting weight gain of 2kg in 3 days. Instead of sending her to A&E (where she might wait 12 hours and risk infection), the specialist nurse books her into the AHFU for the next morning. She receives IV diuretics, her weight drops by 1.5kg, and she sleeps in her own bed that night.

3. Virtual Wards and "Hospital at Home"

The most significant shift in the 2025/26 NHS operational guidance is the Virtual Ward. This is not just a phone call; it is a clinical environment.

Tech-Enabled Care: Patients are discharged early with wearable patches monitoring heart rate, respiratory rate, and oxygen saturation.

The "Daily Huddle": As the leader, you start your day not on a physical ward, but looking at a dashboard of 50 patients at home. AI flags the 3 patients who are deteriorating.

Governance: You retain clinical responsibility for these patients. If a patient deteriorates, you must have a "rapid re-entry" pathway that bypasses A&E.

4. Reducing Readmissions: The "Warm Handoff"

Readmissions often happen because the baton is dropped between the hospital cardiologist and the community heart failure nurse.

The "Reach-In" Model: Community nurses should "reach in" to the hospital before discharge, meeting the patient at the bedside to establish a relationship.

Discharge Checklist 2026: No patient leaves without:

A follow-up appointment booked (not just "requested").

An NT-proBNP trajectory.

A supply of "rescue diuretics" and instructions on when to use them.

Part 2: Advanced Diagnostics and Cardiomyopathies (Subtopic 13.2)

Moving from how we organize care to what we diagnose. The era of labeling patients simply as "Heart Failure" is over. We must now identify the specific phenotype. The 2026 curriculum requires "Precision Phenotyping."
1. Cardiac Magnetic Resonance (CMR) – The Gold Standard

Echocardiography remains the workhorse, but CMR is the "truth machine" for tissue characterization. You must move beyond just looking at the Ejection Fraction (EF).

Tissue Characterization (LGE and T1 Mapping)

Late Gadolinium Enhancement (LGE): This tells us about scarring.

Ischaemic Pattern: Sub-endocardial scar (follows coronary territory).

Non-Ischaemic Pattern: Mid-wall striae (classic in Dilated Cardiomyopathy - DCM).

T1 Mapping: Crucial for diffuse disease.

Scenario: A patient with normal wall thickness but breathlessness. High T1 values might suggest early inflammation or diffuse fibrosis before LGE appears.

Diagnostic Example: A 35-year-old male presents with syncope and a "normal" echo. A CMR is ordered. It reveals a specific "ring-like" sub-epicardial LGE pattern. This serves as a red flag for Arrhythmogenic Left Ventricular Cardiomyopathy (ALVC), a diagnosis completely missed by echo. This changes the plan from reassurance to genetic testing and potential ICD implantation.

2. Nuclear Scintigraphy and the Amyloid Revolution

Amyloidosis (specifically ATTR-CM) was once considered rare. In 2026, we know it is a common cause of HFpEF (Heart Failure with preserved Ejection Fraction) in the elderly.

The "Bone Scan" (Tc-99m DPD/PYP) You must be expert in interpreting these scans. The tracer binds to calcium in the amyloid deposits.

Perugini Grading:

Grade 0: No uptake (Negative).

Grade 2/3: Strong uptake (Positive for ATTR amyloidosis).

The Trap: AL Amyloidosis (a haematological emergency) can also show mild uptake. Therefore, you must always rule out light chains (blood/urine tests) before confirming ATTR.

Clinical Scenario: A 75-year-old man with "thick heart walls" is assumed to have hypertensive heart disease. However, he is hypotensive (low BP) and has Carpal Tunnel Syndrome (a key red flag). You order a DPD scan. It lights up (Grade 3). You diagnose Wild-Type ATTR Amyloidosis and start him on Tafamidis (or newer gene silencers available in 2026), halting the disease.

3. Endomyocardial Biopsy (EMB)

While imaging has reduced the need for biopsy, the advanced trainee must know when to be invasive.

Indications:

Fulminant Myocarditis: Young patient, rapid crash, need to rule out Giant Cell Myocarditis (which needs aggressive immunosuppression).

Storage Diseases: If MRI/Genetic testing is inconclusive for suspected Fabry or Sarcoidosis.

The Procedure: It is high risk. Leadership means knowing when not to do it, just as much as when to do it.

4. Cardiomyopathies and Family Screening

Managing cardiomyopathies is effectively managing a family tree, not just a patient.

Hypertrophic Cardiomyopathy (HCM)

Risk Stratification: We use the "HCM Risk-SCD Calculator."

New Therapies: In 2026, cardiac myosin inhibitors (like Mavacamten) are standard for obstructive HCM, often delaying or cancelling the need for septal reduction surgery.

Dilated Cardiomyopathy (DCM)

Genetics: We now know that specific genes (e.g., Lamin A/C or Filamin C) carry a massive arrhythmia risk even if the pumping function is only mildly reduced.

The "Gene-First" Approach: If you find a Lamin A/C mutation, you might implant a defibrillator (ICD) much earlier than in a standard DCM patient.

Family Screening Coordination

The Cascade: Once a "Proband" (first affected family member) is identified, you must coordinate screening for all first-degree relatives.

The Clinic: This requires a dedicated "Inherited Cardiac Conditions (ICC)" clinic. It is unethical to mix these healthy, anxious relatives with sick acute HF patients in a general clinic.

Validation Point: A young woman dies suddenly. Post-mortem shows ARVC (Arrhythmogenic Right Ventricular Cardiomyopathy). As the leader, you do not close the file. You bring in her parents and siblings. You screen them with ECG, Holter, and MRI. You find her brother has the same early signs. You treat him, likely saving his life. This is the ultimate "preventative" leadership.

13.3 Cardio-Oncology and Specialist Conditions

In the UK, the Cardio-Oncology service has evolved from a niche interest into a mandatory pillar of the Advanced Heart Failure curriculum. Why? Because cancer and heart failure are the two competing giants of morbidity in the Western world. When they collide, the patient is often left stranded between an oncologist who fears stopping the cure and a cardiologist who fears the cure is lethal.

A. The Multi-Specialty MDT: The Art of Negotiation

The curriculum explicitly demands participation in the Cardio-Oncology MDT. This is not a passive lecture; it is a negotiation table.

Imagine a 45-year-old woman with HER2-positive breast cancer. Her tumour is curable, but her LVEF has dropped from 55% to 40% on Trastuzumab.

The Oncologist's Fear: "If we stop, the cancer returns."

The Cardiologist's Fear: "If we continue, she develops irreversible heart failure."

Your role in the MDT is to interpret the risk. In 2026, we move away from the binary "stop/go" mentality. Instead, we use "permissive cardiotoxicity"—supporting the heart aggressively with SGLT2 inhibitors and beta-blockers to allow the cancer treatment to finish. You must learn to speak the language of oncology: understanding the difference between the irreversible Type 1 toxicity of Anthracyclines (like Doxorubicin) and the largely reversible Type 2 toxicity of Trastuzumab.

Clinical Insight:

You will often see patients on Immune Checkpoint Inhibitors (ICIs) like Pembrolizumab. While these drugs are revolutionary for melanoma and lung cancer, they can trigger fulminant myocarditis. This is not the slow drift of heart failure; it is an electrical storm. In the MDT, your job is to recognize the triad of elevated Troponin, conduction block on ECG, and preserved function on Echo—and advocate for immediate high-dose steroids.

B. HF with Pulmonary Hypertension (PH-LHD): The Hemodynamic Puzzle

The second half of subtopic 13.3 focuses on the "wet lung" phenotype. Most Pulmonary Hypertension (PH) you see is Group 2—caused by the failing left heart pushing pressure back into the lungs.

However, the curriculum requires you to master the Right Heart Catheterization (RHC) to distinguish between:

Isolated Post-Capillary PH (Ipc-PH): The lungs are just victims of the left heart. The Diastolic Pressure Gradient (DPG) is low (<7 mmHg), and Pulmonary Vascular Resistance (PVR) is normal. Treatment: Fix the left heart (diuretics, valve repair).

Combined Pre- and Post-Capillary PH (Cpc-PH): The "reactive" lung. The pressure has been high for so long that the pulmonary arteries have clamped down/remodeled. The PVR is elevated (>2-3 Wood Units).

Why does this matter? If you misdiagnose Cpc-PH as simple heart failure, you might miss the fact that this patient is becoming ineligible for a heart transplant (because a new heart cannot pump against those stiff lungs—it would fail immediately in the theatre). Conversely, if you mistake it for PAH (Group 1), you might dangerously prescribe vasodilators like Sildenafil, which can flood the left ventricle and cause pulmonary edema in these patients. Your interpretation of the RHC traces is the safety net.

13.4 Transplantation and Mechanical Support (MCS)

This subtopic represents the "end of the road" for standard therapy. When the medications fail and the defib shocks become frequent, we look to the tertiary options: replacement or support.

A. The Gatekeeper: Assessment for Transplant & LVAD

Identifying the patient for tertiary therapy is an exercise in timing. Refer too early, and you subject a stable patient to unnecessary surgical risk. Refer too late, and the "window of opportunity" closes as end-organ dysfunction (kidney/liver failure) sets in.

You must become proficient in interpreting the Cardiopulmonary Exercise Test (CPET). This is the ultimate stress test.

The Magic Number: A Peak VO2 of <12-14 ml/kg/min is the traditional cut-off where the risk of staying on medical therapy exceeds the risk of transplant.

The VE/VCO2 Slope: If this is >35, it indicates inefficient ventilation and poor prognosis, even if the VO2 looks borderline.

The "Soft" Intelligence: The curriculum emphasizes psychosocial assessment. A heart transplant is not a cure; it is a trade-off of one chronic disease (heart failure) for another (immunosuppression). You must assess the patient's "medical adherence." Do they attend appointments? do they have a support network? A brilliant surgical outcome can be ruined in weeks if a patient forgets their Tacrolimus.

B. Mechanical Circulatory Support (LVAD): The Modern Cyborg

In the UK context (2026), the Left Ventricular Assist Device (LVAD) is primarily used as a Bridge to Transplant (BTT), though functionally many patients remain on it for years (Bridge to Candidacy or Destination Therapy).

The modern LVAD (like the HeartMate 3) is a magnetically levitated centrifugal pump. It is continuous flow—meaning your patient will not have a pulse.

BP Management: You cannot use a standard cuff. You need a Doppler probe to find the "opening pressure" (MAP), targeting 70-80 mmHg. High pressure causes stroke; low pressure causes pump thrombosis.

The Driveline: This cable exiting the abdomen is the Achilles' heel. It is a direct highway for bacteria (Staph aureus) to enter the sterile pump pocket. As a trainee, you must inspect the exit site with the vigilance of a hawk. A red,crusty driveline exit site is a medical emergency.

C. The Transplanted Patient: Shared Care and Surveillance

Once the patient receives a heart, the physiology changes. The donor heart is denervated—the vagus nerve is cut.

Physiological quirk: Atropine doesn't work on a transplant heart (no vagal input to block). If they are bradycardic, you need Isoprenaline or pacing. Angina is rare because they can't feel chest pain; ischemia presents as "silent" breathlessness or fatigue.

Rejection Surveillance: You will manage the schedule of Endomyocardial Biopsies.

Cellular Rejection: T-lymphocytes attack the myocardium. The biopsy shows infiltration. We treat with high-dose steroids/ATG.

Antibody-Mediated Rejection (AMR): B-cells create antibodies against the donor HLA. This is harder to treat (requires Plasmapheresis/Rituximab) and carries a worse prognosis.

Deep Dive Analysis: The "2026" Perspective

As of today, January 2026, the landscape has shifted slightly from the old textbooks.

1. The "Pre-Symptomatic" Toxicity Detection: We no longer wait for the Ejection Fraction to drop. In Cardio-Oncology, we rely heavily on Global Longitudinal Strain (GLS). A drop in GLS of >15% is an early warning siren, sounding months before the EF changes. This allows us to start "cardioprotection" (ACEi/Beta-blockers) invisibly, keeping the patient on their life-saving chemotherapy.

2. The Xenotransplant Horizon: While still experimental, the conversations in 2025/2026 around pig-heart xenotransplantation are growing. As an advanced trainee, while you won't be doing this routinely, you must be conversant in the ethics and the emerging immunology of this field, as it represents the only scalable solution to the donor organ shortage.

3. The Rise of Amyloid: A crucial part of the "Specialist Conditions" in 2026 is the explosion in diagnosing Transthyretin Amyloidosis (ATTR). We now have drugs (Tafamidis, Silencers) that treat this. In your transplant assessment, you must rigorously screen for Amyloid (using DPD bone scans) because these patients have specific needs—they often don't tolerate standard HF meds (beta-blockers/ACEi) due to autonomic neuropathy and small, stiff ventricles.

2. Simulation and Foundation Skills (Subtopic 14.1)

2.1 The Pre-Patient Requirement

Subtopic 14.1 establishes a non-negotiable barrier: procedural skill acquisition must begin before the patient encounter. This is a profound ethical and educational stance. It acknowledges that the learning curve for invasive procedures carries inherent risks—bleeding, perforation, infection, or arrhythmia. To mitigate these risks, the curriculum mandates "Skills Lab" training.

In the context of 2026, simulation is not just about playing with plastic mannequins. It involves high-fidelity haptic feedback systems that mimic the resistance of human tissue.

Example: Consider the procedure of temporary pacing. In a skills lab, a trainee can practice inserting a pacing wire into a mannequin's jugular vein. If they puncture the simulated carotid artery, the system flashes a warning. The trainee learns to recognize the angle of the needle and the tactile "pop" of entering the vein without endangering a human life. This creates a "safe failure" environment where mistakes become learning points, not clinical incidents.

2.2 The "Big Three" Simulated Procedures

The curriculum specifically highlights three procedures that require this simulation-first approach:

Temporary Pacing: This involves placing an electrical wire into the heart to maintain a heartbeat during bradycardia (slow heart rate). It requires understanding venous anatomy and electrical thresholds.

Pericardiocentesis: This is the drainage of fluid from the sac surrounding the heart. It is a high-risk procedure because the needle passes millimeters from the coronary arteries and the right ventricle.

DC Cardioversion: This involves delivering an electric shock to reset the heart's rhythm. While less invasive than needles, it requires perfect synchronization and airway management.

2.3 The Triad of Foundational Safety

Beyond the mechanical skills, Subtopic 14.1 emphasizes three pillars of safety that must be mastered in simulation before touching a patient. These are often called "non-technical skills," but they are just as vital as manual dexterity.

Aseptic Technique: Infection is a devastating complication in cardiology. Devices like pacemakers are foreign bodies; if bacteria colonize them, they create biofilms that are impossible to treat with antibiotics alone.

Deep Dive: In simulation, trainees practice the ritual of scrubbing, gowning, and draping. They learn to create a "sterile field" where nothing unsterile can enter. This muscle memory ensures that when they are in a stressful emergency, they do not accidentally break sterility.

Safe Sedation: Many cardiology procedures are uncomfortable. Cardiologists must administer sedative drugs (like midazolam or fentanyl) to keep the patient calm.

Deep Dive: The danger is "oversedation," where the patient stops breathing. Simulation training involves managing a "simulated patient" whose oxygen levels drop. The trainee must learn to titrate the drug carefully—giving enough for comfort, but not so much that the airway is compromised.

Valid Consent: This is the legal and ethical foundation of medicine. Before a knife touches skin, the patient must understand the risks.

Deep Dive: Trainees role-play the consent conversation. They must explain complex risks (e.g., "There is a 1% chance of puncturing the lung") in simple language to an actor playing a frightened patient. This verifies that the trainee truly understands the procedure well enough to explain it simply.

Only once a trainee has demonstrated competence in these simulated domains can they progress to Level 2 (Supervised Clinical Practice), where they perform the procedure on a real patient under the direct, unblinking observation of a mentor.

3. Core Procedural Competencies (Subtopic 14.2)

3.1 Defining "Competence" (The Levels)

To understand Subtopic 14.2, we must first define the language of competency levels used in UK medical training.

Level 1: Theory and observation only.

Level 2: Supervised practice (the trainer is scrubbed in next to you).

Level 3: Indirect supervision (the trainer is in the room or nearby, available immediately).

Level 4: Unsupervised competence. The trainee can perform the procedure independently and handle common complications.

Subtopic 14.2 details the journey to Level 4 for "Core Procedures." These are the skills that every consultant cardiologist must possess, regardless of their sub-specialty. Whether you end up specializing in heart failure or imaging, you must be able to put in a central line or pace a heart in an emergency.

3.2 Analysis of Table 14.1: The Progression Matrix

The table provided in the curriculum outlines a specific timeline for skill acquisition. We will analyze this by procedure to understand the logic behind the progression.

4. Deep Dive Analysis: The "Early Mastery" Group (ST4 Targets)

The curriculum dictates that by the end of ST4 (Specialty Training Year 4—the first year of specialized cardiology training), a registrar must already be at Level 4 (independent) for several key procedures. These are the bread-and-butter skills of acute hospital care.

4.1 Central Venous Cannulation (CVC) & Arterial Lines

Requirement: Level 4 at ST4.

Why so early? These are critical care skills. Patients with heart attacks or heart failure often need potent drugs that cannot go through small arm veins. They need a "Central Line" in the neck (internal jugular vein) or groin (femoral vein). Similarly, they need continuous blood pressure monitoring via an "Arterial Line" in the wrist.

The Procedure: The trainee uses ultrasound guidance—a standard of care in 2026. They visualize the vein, ensuring it is patent (open) and not clotted. They guide a needle into the vessel, feed a wire through the needle, and then slide a plastic tube (catheter) over the wire. This is known as the Seldinger Technique.

Clinical Relevance: If a patient enters the Cardiac Intensive Care Unit (CICU) in shock, the registrar cannot wait for a supervisor. They must establish access immediately to deliver life-saving vasopressors (drugs that raise blood pressure). This explains why Level 4 is required immediately at ST4.

4.2 DC Cardioversion (DCCV)

Requirement: Level 4 at ST4.

The Procedure: This is used for Atrial Fibrillation (an irregular heart rhythm). The doctor applies pads to the patient's chest and back. They synchronize the defibrillator to the patient's R-wave (the peak of the heartbeat) to avoid causing cardiac arrest.

Why so early? DCCV is one of the most common procedures in cardiology. It is performed daily for elective patients and urgently for unstable patients. An ST4 registrar is often the "senior" doctor on the ward at night; they must be able to shock a patient back into a normal rhythm without calling a consultant from home.

4.3 Emergency Echocardiography

Requirement: Level 4 at ST4.

Distinction: Note the difference between "Emergency Echo" and "Transthoracic Echo." Emergency Echo is a focused scan. The question is simple: "Is there fluid around the heart? Is the heart pumping at all? Is the right side of the heart swollen?"

Clinical Relevance: In a cardiac arrest or profound shock, a full diagnostic scan takes too long. The registrar needs to grab the probe and get a "Yes/No" answer in seconds. This saves lives, which is why independence is required from the very start of training.

5. Deep Dive Analysis: The "gradual Mastery" Group

For higher-risk or more complex procedures, the curriculum allows a slower maturation process, moving from the Skills Lab at ST4 to full independence at the end of training (ST8).

5.1 Temporary Pacing

Progression: Skills Lab (ST4) → Level 3 (ST6) → Level 4 (ST8).

The Complexity: Temporary pacing is significantly harder than putting in a central line. The doctor must not only enter the vein but also float a wire blindly through the heart chambers, across the tricuspid valve, and lodge it into the muscle of the right ventricle.

The Risk: If the wire goes too far, it can puncture the heart (tamponade). If it doesn't touch the wall firmly, it won't capture the rhythm, and the patient's heart will stop.

The Learning Curve:

ST4: The trainee learns the mechanics on a simulator.

ST6: The trainee performs the procedure on patients but with a consultant in the room (Level 3). This is crucial because complications happen quickly.

ST8: The trainee is now a master. They can do it alone at 3 AM. This gradual release of responsibility ensures patient safety during the steep learning curve.

5.2 Pericardiocentesis

Progression: Skills Lab (ST4) → Level 3 (ST6) → Level 4 (ST8).

The Stakes: This is perhaps the most daunting core procedure. It involves pushing a long needle towards a beating heart to drain fluid (pericardial effusion) that is crushing the heart chambers.

Why Level 4 at CCT? This condition (Cardiac Tamponade) is a medical emergency. If a patient collapses with tamponade, they will die before a surgeon can arrive. Therefore, every graduating cardiologist must be able to relieve the pressure with a needle. However, because the procedure is rare and dangerous, it takes years (from ST4 to ST8) to accumulate enough supervised cases to be truly safe.

5.3 Transthoracic Echocardiography (TTE)

Progression: Level 2 (ST4) → Level 4 (ST6).

The Skill: Unlike "Emergency Echo," this is a full diagnostic study. It involves taking precise measurements of valve flow, pressure gradients, and chamber volumes.

The Timeline: It takes hundreds of hours of scanning to develop the "eye-brain" coordination to spot subtle defects. By ST6, a registrar is expected to report these scans independently, acting as a definitive diagnostic resource for the hospital.

6. The Role of Maintenance

A crucial aspect of Table 14.1 is the column labeled "Maintain." Once a trainee reaches Level 4 (e.g., for Central Lines at ST4), they are not finished. They must maintain that skill for the next four years.

The Decay of Skills: Procedural skills degrade if not used. A registrar who masters cardioversion in ST4 but never does another one until ST8 will become unsafe. The curriculum mandates continuous engagement. This might mean keeping a logbook where the registrar records a minimum number of procedures annually to prove they haven't lost their touch.

Example: An ST7 registrar (nearly a consultant) might be focusing heavily on MRI or genetics. However, if they are on-call for the general cardiology ward, they must still be able to insert a temporary pacing wire. The "Maintain" requirement ensures they remain a "generalist" even as they become a "specialist."

7. Integration of Technology and Future Outlook (2026)

Writing this from the perspective of 2026, we can see how technology aids these curriculum requirements.

Ultrasound for Everything: By 2026, "blind" landmark techniques are obsolete. The curriculum implies that all vascular access and pericardiocentesis are done under real-time ultrasound guidance. This visual confirmation drastically reduces complications.

Virtual Reality (VR): The "Skills Lab" mentioned in 14.1 increasingly utilizes VR headsets. This allows trainees to practice the "steps" of a procedure mentally—visualizing the equipment tray, the hand movements, and the teamwork—before entering the physical lab.

Procedure Specific Assessment (DOPS): In the UK system, competence is verified through assessments called DOPS (Direct Observation of Procedural Skills). A trainee cannot just say "I can do it." They must submit forms where a consultant verifies, "I watched Dr. X perform this pericardiocentesis; their aseptic technique was perfect, they recognized the anatomy, and the patient remained stable."

Section 1: Advanced Procedural Divergence (Subtopic 14.3)

1.1 The Philosophy of Divergence

The concept of "Procedural Divergence" is the structural backbone of the ST6-ST8 years. In the past, there was often an unspoken pressure for all cardiologists to be "jacks of all trades," dabbling in complex pacing or angioplasty. The current curriculum recognizes that this is no longer safe or feasible.

Divergence ensures that training time is efficient. A trainee destined for a career in Heart Failure or Imaging does not need to spend precious hours refining complex wire manipulation for angioplasty; they need just enough skill to be safe and diagnostic. Conversely, the Interventional trainee must sacrifice breadth in other areas to achieve the extreme dexterity required for Level 4 competence.

This divergence relies on the "Level 3 vs. Level 4" entrustment scale:

Level 3 (Indirect Supervision): The trainee can perform the procedure. The consultant is in the building but not in the room. This is the standard for the Generalist.

Level 4 (Unsupervised): The trainee acts independently, capable of dealing with complex anatomy and complications without immediate backup. This is the standard for the Specialist.

1.2 Case Study: Diagnostic Coronary Angiography (DCA)

Nowhere is divergence more visible than in the cath lab.

The Generalist Requirement (Level 3): For the general cardiology trainee, the goal of DCA is diagnostic certainty and safety. By ST6, the generalist must demonstrate the ability to engage native coronary arteries and bypass grafts (LIMA/veins) safely. Their focus is on:

Vascular Access: Proficient radial access (and safe femoral conversion if required).

Hemodynamics: Accurate pressure recording (LVEDP).

Interpretation: Recognizing "critical" vs. "non-critical" disease to facilitate referral.

Example: A Heart Failure trainee performing an angiogram on a dilated cardiomyopathy patient needs to rule out ischemic causes. If they encounter a tortuous subclavian artery, they may ask for help. This is acceptable for Level 3. Their competence is defined by knowing their limit.

The Interventional Trainee Requirement (Level 4): For the trainee in the Interventional theme, Level 3 is merely a stepping stone. By ST6/ST7, they must operate at Level 4. This involves a different cognitive and manual skill set:

Complex Anatomy: The ability to navigate extreme tortuosity, anomalous take-offs, or calcified vessels without causing dissection.

Support: Understanding guide catheter support (active vs. passive) which is a precursor to PCI (Percutaneous Coronary Intervention).

Efficiency: Performing the procedure with minimal contrast load and radiation dose, preserving physiological reserve for potential immediate intervention.

Example: The Interventional trainee encounters the same tortuous subclavian. They are expected to use advanced maneuver techniques (e.g., balloon-assisted tracking or long sheaths) to overcome the anatomy independently. Calling for help for "routine" complexity is a marker of not yet achieving Level 4.

1.3 Case Study: Permanent Pacemaker Implantation (PPM)

The Generalist Requirement (Level 3): The "General Cardiology" curriculum demands competence in bradycardia pacing. This is a safety net for the NHS; any consultant cardiologist on call should be able to temporarily pace a patient or, in many centers, implant a straightforward dual-chamber system for complete heart block.

Scope: Standard right ventricular and right atrial lead placement.

Troubleshooting: Basic threshold management and sensing issues.

Example: An elderly patient presents with syncope and Complete Heart Block. The generalist trainee (Level 3) is expected to safely implant a dual-chamber PPM. If the subclavian vein is inaccessible, they might defer to a specialist or call for senior help.

The Arrhythmia Specialist Requirement (Level 4): For the trainee leading an arrhythmia service, the procedural requirement expands exponentially.

Device Complexity: It is not just about "putting a lead in." It involves His-bundle pacing (HBP) or Left Bundle Branch Area Pacing (LBBAP)—techniques that have become standard by 2026 to preserve physiological ventricular function.

Revision & Extraction: Managing infected pockets, upgrading systems (e.g., PPM to CRT), and extracting chronic leads.

Autonomy: The specialist must be able to troubleshoot "displaced leads" or "high thresholds" intra-operatively without scrubbing out to find a consultant.

Section 2: Complication Management (Subtopic 14.4)
2.1 The "Black Swan" in Training

Procedural medicine is defined not by how well one performs when things go right, but by how one reacts when they go wrong. Subtopic 14.4 mandates that complication management is not theoretical; it must be rehearsed, evidenced, and ingrained.

By 2026, the reliance on high-fidelity simulation (HFS) has grown. Trainees often face their first "pericardial tamponade" in a simulator before they face it in a patient. However, the curriculum requires evidence of management in real-world or near-real-world environments.

2.2 Specific Adverse Events & Management Protocols

A. Vascular Access Bleeding & Retroperitoneal Hematoma

The Scenario: A femoral puncture goes high, leading to a retroperitoneal bleed.

Curriculum Requirement: The trainee must demonstrate early recognition (back pain, hypotension without obvious blood loss).

Management: Immediate volume resuscitation, reversal of anticoagulation, and knowing when to call vascular surgery or interventional radiology for balloon tamponade of the iliac artery.

B. Pericardial Tamponade This is the "classic" cath lab nightmare.

Recognition: The trainee must spot the "dipping" pressure trace and the cessation of contrast movement in the pericardial space before the patient arrests.

Action: Emergency pericardiocentesis.

Divergence: A Level 3 generalist must be able to drain the fluid safely. A Level 4 interventionalist might be expected to seal the perforation with a covered stent or balloon while the drain is in situ.

C. Procedural Stroke

The Scenario: Aortic plaque disruption leads to a dense hemiparesis on the table.

Management: This tests "Leadership" more than manual skill. The trainee must immediately coordinate with the stroke team, maintain hemodynamics, and decide on the safety of completing the cardiac procedure versus aborting. By 2026, knowing the local pathway for mechanical thrombectomy is a mandatory curriculum item.

2.3 The Duty of Candour & Human Factors

The 2026 curriculum places a massive emphasis on the post-complication phase. The technical fix is only half the job.

Duty of Candour (Regulation 20): The trainee must demonstrate the ability to have the "difficult conversation" with the family.

Authenticity: It is not about reading a legal script. It is about explaining: "A complication has occurred. We have recognized it. This is what we have done to fix it. This is what it means for your father."

Verification: Trainers assess this via Workplace Based Assessments (CbD - Case-based Discussion) specifically focused on communication ethics.

Team Debriefing: Following a major complication (e.g., a cardiac arrest in the lab), the trainee must lead the "Hot Debrief."

Objective: To ensure team welfare and capture immediate learning points without assigning blame.

Skill: The ability to flatten the hierarchy, allowing the scrub nurse or radiographer to speak up about what they saw. This aligns with the "Just Culture" framework pivotal to NHS safety standards.

Section 3: The Integration of Simulation & Technology (2026 Context)

In 2026, "Advanced Procedural Divergence" is heavily supported by AI-driven simulation.

For the Generalist: Simulation allows them to maintain "competence" in low-volume skills (like temporary pacing) without needing to hunt for rare cases on the wards.

For the Specialist: Patient-specific simulation (using CT-derived 3D models) allows interventional trainees to "practice" a complex TAVI or bifurcation PCI on a digital twin before touching the patient.

This technology bridges the gap between Level 3 and Level 4. It allows trainees to fail safely, repeatedly, until the divergence to expert status is genuine and earned, not just a function of time served.

Assessment, Quality Management, and Recruitment Context

Subtopic 15.1: The European Examination in Core Cardiology (EECC)

1. Overview and Strategic Importance

The EECC is the "Standard Bearer" of knowledge in your training. While your daily work validates your hands, this exam validates your mind. It is a mandatory, summative assessment typically taken during ST5 (the final year of Core Cardiology training under the 2022 curriculum).

Why is it critical? Passing the EECC is a non-negotiable prerequisite for the award of your Certificate of Completion of Training (CCT). In the current 2026 training landscape, it also acts as a "gateway." Failing to pass this exam can arrest your progression into advanced sub-specialty modules (e.g., complex intervention or EP) because it signals a gap in core knowledge.

Authentic Insight: Do not underestimate the breadth of this exam. Many trainees excel in their specific sub-interest (e.g., interventional fellows knowing everything about stents) but fail the EECC because they neglected "cinderella" topics like congenital heart disease, genetics, or pericardial diseases. The EECC demands you be a generalist first.

2. Exam Format and Delivery (2026 Specification)

As per the confirmed schedule for the 2026 academic year, the exam structure remains rigorous and digital-first.

Date: Tuesday, 16 June 2026.

Platform: Online Proctoring (ProctorU). You take this from home or a private office, not a test center.

Duration: 3 hours continuous (no scheduled breaks).

Volume: 120 Multiple Choice Questions (MCQs).

Question Style: "Best of Five." You are given a clinical vignette and five plausible options. You must choose the most appropriate action or diagnosis. Negative marking is not used.

The "UK Twist": Although this is a European exam (harmonized across nations like Germany, Spain, and Italy), UK trainees face a slightly modified version. Your paper will include 6 UK-specific questions. These focus on NICE guidelines or DVLA driving restrictions for cardiac patients—areas where UK legislation differs from general European consensus.

3. The Curriculum: What is Actually Tested?

The exam is blueprint-mapped to the 2020 ESC Core Curriculum. It does not test niche, cutting-edge research that was published last week. It tests established, guideline-driven medicine.

High-Yield Areas include:

Valvular Heart Disease: Timing of surgery (asymptomatic severe Aortic Stenosis).

Heart Failure: The "Four Pillars" of medical therapy and device eligibility (CRT-D/P).

Prevention: Lipid management targets (increasingly aggressive in 2026 guidelines) and hypertension.

Imaging: Interpretation of Echo loops, CMR stills, and basic nuclear cardiology.

Rhythm Disorders: ECG diagnosis (wide complex tachycardia differentiation) and ablation indications.

Figure 15.1: A typical exam stimulus. You might be asked to differentiate VT from SVT with aberrancy based on Brugada criteria.

4. Standard Setting: The Pass Mark

How do you pass? The EECC uses the Hofstee Method (a compromise between absolute and relative standards) to set the pass mark.

Historically, the pass mark hovers between 54% and 58%.

This sounds low, but the questions are highly discriminative.

Result Release: Late July 2026.

5. Strategic Preparation for 2026

The "March Window": Registration usually closes in early 2026. Once registered, you gain access to the ESC Preparatory Course in March 2026. Use this resource. It is the only "official" question bank.

Guidelines over Textbooks: Do not read massive textbooks cover-to-cover. Read the "ESC Guidelines" summaries. If a guideline says "Class I Recommendation," it is fair game for a question.

The Visual Trap: 30% of questions contain images (ECGs, Echo, Angio). If you practice only with text-based MCQs, you will struggle with the cognitive load of interpreting a video loop on a laptop screen under time pressure.

Subtopic 15.2: Workplace-Based Assessments (WPBAs)

If the EECC is the snapshot, WPBAs are the documentary film of your training. Under the 2022 curriculum, the focus of WPBAs shifted from "Assessment of Performance" to "Supervised Learning Events" (SLEs).

The distinction is vital: An SLE is formative. It is a teaching moment. You should not be afraid to trigger a WPBA for a difficult case where you didn't know the answer—that is often the best evidence of learning!
1. ACAT (Acute Care Assessment Tool)

The "Take" Simulator. The ACAT is unique to UK medical training. It does not assess a single patient interaction; it assesses your ability to run the "Acute Take" (the admission of emergency patients).

Requirement: Minimum of 5 cases per ACAT.

Key Competencies:

Prioritization: Who needs the Echo now vs. tomorrow?

Leadership: How do you manage the junior doctors and nursing team during a cardiac arrest?

Handover: The quality of your post-take ward round documentation.

Validating Example:

Scenario: You are the SpR on call. You have a patient with VT in Resus, a STEMI call in the ambulance bay, and a query aortic dissection in minors. An ACAT assessment here observes how you deploy your team. Do you send the SHO to the dissection? Do you go to the STEMI yourself? The ACAT validates your "bandwidth" and safety as a leader, not just your medical knowledge.

2. CbD (Case-Based Discussion)

The Deep Dive into Logic. The CbD is a retrospective look at your decision-making. It usually involves selecting a case you have managed and sitting down with a consultant to critique your notes and letters.

Focus: Clinical reasoning, medical knowledge, and ethical decision-making.

Best Use Case: Complex patients with competing comorbidities (e.g., managing NSTEMI in a patient with active GI bleeding).

2026 Tip: In the modern curriculum, use CbDs to tick off "CiPs" (Capabilities in Practice) related to outpatient clinics. Discussing a complex clinic letter you wrote is often higher yield than discussing an acute admission.

3. DOPS (Direct Observation of Procedural Skills)

The "Licence to Operate". Cardiology is a craft specialty. DOPS are the evidence that your hands are safe. In 2026, the scrutiny on procedural safety is higher than ever.

Critical DOPS Requirements (2022 Curriculum):

Diagnostic Angiography: You must demonstrate competency in both radial and femoral access.

Pacing: Temporary pacing is a dying art but a mandatory skill. You need 6 DOPS total, with at least one Level 5 (Independent) performed in the final two years of training.

Pericardiocentesis: A rare but life-saving skill. You need 4 DOPS. Crucially, simulation is accepted for 3 of these, but you must have at least one on a real patient or a high-fidelity 'wet' model assessed at Level 5.

Figure 15.2: Ultrasound guidance for femoral access is now a standard of care. A DOPS assessment here checks your ability to maintain sterility while operating the probe and needle simultaneously.

The Grading Scale:

Level 3: Needs direct supervision (Trainer in the room, scrubbed).

Level 4: Needs indirect supervision (Trainer in the room, unscrubbed).

Level 5: Independent (Trainer can be having coffee nearby).

4. MCR (Multiple Consultant Report)

The Holistic Verdict. The MCR is arguably the most powerful tool in the 2026 arsenal. It replaces the singular opinion of one supervisor with the "wisdom of the crowd."

Mechanism: Twice a year (usually), all the consultants you work with receive a digital form. They rate you against the "CiPs" (e.g., "Is this trainee safe to run the unselected take?").

The Power of Narrative: The text boxes in an MCR are more important than the scores. A comment like "I would happily let Dr. X treat my father" is the gold standard of validation. Conversely, "Technically gifted but abrasive with nursing staff" will trigger a remedial meeting.

Minimum Requirement: For Cardiology, you generally require 4 Consultant responses per MCR cycle to be considered valid for your ARCP (Annual Review of Competence Progression).

Deep Dive Analysis: The Integration of Assessment

How do these two subtopics (EECC and WPBAs) interact? They form the X and Y axes of your competence graph.

The Knowledge-Skill Gap: It is possible to pass the EECC (High Knowledge) but fail your DOPS (Low Skill). This creates a "Technician" profile—someone who knows the guidelines but cannot safely deploy a stent.

The Dangerous Operator: Conversely, a trainee with excellent hands (Level 5 DOPS) who fails the EECC (Low Knowledge) is dangerous. They can perform the procedure perfectly, but they may be doing it on the wrong patient because they didn't understand the guidelines.

The ARCP Panel's View in 2026: When your panel meets in June/July 2026, they will look for concordance.

Does the CbD evidence support the knowledge shown in the EECC?

Does the MCR feedback on "teamworking" align with the leadership skills shown in the ACAT?

15.3 The ARCP Process and Critical Progression Points

The Annual Review of Competence Progression (ARCP) is not merely a box-ticking exercise; it is the statutory mechanism that ratifies a doctor's ability to hold a National Training Number (NTN). In the 2022 curriculum (fully operational for all trainees in 2026), the ARCP focuses less on time served and more on the acquisition of Capabilities in Practice (CiPs).

The ARCP Decision Aid: The "Matrix" of Progression

The "ARCP Decision Aid" is the definitive document used by panels to determine if a trainee can progress to the next year. It removes ambiguity by setting specific, numerical targets for workplace-based assessments (WPBAs). For a trainee moving through Core Cardiology (ST4 and ST5), the targets are rigorous.

Key Decision Aid Targets (ST4/ST5):

Supervised Learning Events (SLEs): Trainees must complete a minimum of 5 Case-based Discussions (CbD) or Mini-Clinical Evaluation Exercises (mini-CEX) per year. These are not just "pass/fail" events; they must demonstrate high-quality feedback from consultants.

Acute Care Assessment Tool (ACAT): A minimum of 3 ACATs per year is required. Each ACAT must cover at least 5 cases, assessing the trainee's ability to run the "acute take"—a critical skill for the dual-accreditation (GIM) component.

Multi-Source Feedback (MSF): A robust MSF with at least 12 raters, including 3 consultants, is mandatory. This ensures that "soft skills" like teamwork and leadership are scrutinised alongside clinical acumen.

The "High-Stakes" Practical Procedures: The Decision Aid also mandates specific procedural competencies. For instance, by the end of core training, a trainee must have:

Temporary Pacing: 6 DOPS (Direct Observation of Procedural Skills), with at least 3 at "Level 5" (competent to perform independently).

Pericardiocentesis: 4 DOPS, with at least 1 at "Level 5."

Analysis: The specificity of the Decision Aid protects the trainee. If a trainee has met these numbers, an ARCP panel cannot arbitrarily delay them. Conversely, it protects the public; a trainee without these specific sign-offs cannot proceed, regardless of how "good" they seem on the ward.

The Critical Progression Point (ST5 to ST6)

The most significant hurdle in the curriculum is the Critical Progression Point at the end of ST5. This is the "watershed" moment where the trainee transitions from a generalist "Core Cardiologist" to a specialist in an Advanced Theme (e.g., Interventional Cardiology, Electrophysiology, or Imaging).

Why is it "Critical"? At this junction, the ARCP panel is making a binding decision on the trainee's aptitude for higher-level practice.

Gateway to Specialisation: Entry into ST6 is conditional on having passed the European Exam in Core Cardiology (EECC) (often taken in ST5) and achieving specific CiP entrustment levels (typically Level 3: "Entrusted to act with indirect supervision").

Redirecting Pathways: If a trainee fails to meet the requirements at this point, they cannot simply "drift" into ST6. They may be given an Outcome 3 (extension of training time) to remediate. If they fail again, they may be redirected away from their chosen advanced theme or released from the programme entirely.

Example Scenario: Consider "Dr. A," an ST5 trainee. Dr. A is excellent at echocardiography but has avoided the catheter lab due to anxiety.

Result: At the Critical Progression Point, Dr. A lacks the mandatory "Diagnostic Angiography" sign-offs required for core competence.

Outcome: The ARCP panel cannot allow Dr. A to progress to ST6 (even if they want to be an imaging specialist) because the core curriculum requires angiography competence. Dr. A receives an extension.

15.4 Quality Management and the 2026 Recruitment Framework

While ARCP manages those inside the system, Subtopic 15.4 deals with the rigorous quality assurance of the programme itself and the gateway for new entrants.
Quality Management: The JRCPTB's Watchful Eye

The Joint Royal Colleges of Physicians Training Board (JRCPTB) does not just set the curriculum; it polices it. Quality management is achieved through a triangulation of data:

GMC National Training Surveys: Every year, trainees anonymously rate their posts. If a specific hospital consistently gets "red flags" for inadequate supervision or bullying, the JRCPTB can trigger a "Quality Visit."

About Author

Azhar ul Haque Sario is a bestselling author and data scientist with a remarkable record of achievement. This Cambridge alumnus brings a wealth of knowledge to his work, holding an MBA (SZABIST), ACCA (Knowledge Level - FTMS College Malaysia and London College of Accountancy, London), BBA, and several Google certifications, including specializations in Google Data Analytics, Google Digital Marketing & E-commerce, and Google Project Management.

With ten years of business experience, Azhar combines practical expertise with his impressive academic background to craft insightful books. His prolific writing has resulted in an astounding 2810 published titles, earning him the record for the maximum Kindle editions and paperback books published by an individual author in one year, awarded by Asia Books of Records in 2024.

ORCID: https://orcid.org/0009-0004-8629-830X
Azhar.sario@hotmail.co.uk
https://www.linkedin.com/in/azharulhaquesario/

www.ingramcontent.com/pod-product-compliance
Lightning Source LLC
Chambersburg PA
CBHW031346230926
51848CB00002B/414
9783384808776